THE
BLACK
DOCTORS
OF
COLONIAL LIMA

McGill-Queen's/Associated Medical Services Studies in the History of Medicine, Health, and Society

Series Editors: S.O. Freedman and J.T.H. Connor

Volumes in this series have financial support from Associated Medical Services, Inc. (AMS). Associated Medical Services Inc. was established in 1936 by Dr Jason Hannah as a pioneer prepaid not-for-profit health care organization in Ontario. With the advent of medicare, AMS became a charitable organization supporting innovations in academic medicine and health services, specifically the history of medicine and health care, as well as innovations in health professional education and bioethics.

THE
BLACK
DOCTORS
OF
COLONIAL LIMA

SCIENCE, RACE, and WRITING
in COLONIAL and EARLY
REPUBLICAN PERU

JOSÉ R. JOUVE MARTÍN

McGill-Queen's University Press
Montreal & Kingston • London • Ithaca

© McGill-Queen's University Press 2014

ISBN 978-0-7735-4341-6 (cloth)
ISBN 978-0-7735-9052-6 (ePDF)
ISBN 978-0-7735-9053-3 (ePUB)

Legal deposit second quarter 2014
Bibliothèque nationale du Québec

Printed in Canada on acid-free paper that is 100% ancient forest free
(100% post-consumer recycled), processed chlorine free

McGill-Queen's University Press acknowledges the support of the
Canada Council for the Arts for our publishing program. We also
acknowledge the financial support of the Government of Canada
through the Canada Book Fund for our publishing activities.

Library and Archives Canada Cataloguing in Publication

Jouve Martín, José Ramón, author
The black doctors of colonial Lima : science, race, and writing in
colonial and early Republican Peru / José R. Jouve Martín.

(McGill-Queen's/Associated Medical Services studies in the history
of medicine, health, and society ; 41)
Includes bibliographical references and index.
Issued in print and electronic formats.
ISBN 978-0-7735-4341-6 (bound).–ISBN 978-0-7735-9052-6 (ePDF).
–ISBN 978-0-7735-9053-3 (ePUB)

1. Medicine–Social aspects–Peru–Lima–History. 2. Science–Social
aspects–Peru–Lima–History. 3. Medical writing–Social aspects–
Peru–Lima–History. 4. Race–Social aspects–Peru–Lima–History.
5. Larrinaga, José Pastor, approximately 1750–1823. 6. Dávalos,
José Manuel, 1758–1821. 7. Valdés, José Manuel, 1767–1843. 8.
Physicians–Peru–Lima–History. 9. Surgeons–Peru–Lima–History. 10.
Blacks–Peru–Lima–History. 11. Lima (Peru)–Race relations–History.
12. Peru–Colonization–History. I. Title. II. Series: McGill-Queen's/
Associated Medical Services studies in the history of medicine, health,
and society ; 41

R482.P4J69 2014   610.985   C2013-908518-1
C2013-908519-X

This book was designed and typeset by studio oneonone
in Sabon 10.2/13.5

~

Contents

~

Illustrations

~

Acknowledgments

This book has been made possible thanks to the support of many individuals and institutions. I am indebted to the Canadian Social Sciences and Humanities Research Council (SSHRC) and the Fonds québécois de recherche sur la société et la culture (FQRSC), which supported this research through its generous grant programs. I am also grateful to the Centro superior de investigaciones científicas (CSIC, Spain) and to Alfredo Alvar Ezquerra, for allowing me to be part of his research group La escritura del recuerdo en primera persona (HAR2011-30251). This book has benefited significantly from the commentaries and suggestions made by the external reviewers as well as by Jacqueline Mason, in-house editor at McGill-Queen's University Press. I sincerely thank them for helping me focus and rethink my work. I had a great time working with John Pleasants and Douglas Herrick, who helped me translate and edit important sections of this book. Carlotta Lemieux's extraordinary attention to detail further improved the original text. I have tested the patience of the staff of the Interlibrary Loan Department of McLennan Library at McGill University. They have always been extraordinarily kind and efficient in trying to obtain for me almost everything I requested. I am grateful to the Archivo arzobispal de Lima, the Archivo general de la nación, the Biblioteca nacional de Perú, and all the other Peruvian and Spanish archival repositories that I have worked with, for their guidance and help in obtaining the documents that appear in this monograph. A special thanks to Jesús Pérez-Magallón for his support as a colleague and friend ever since I arrived at McGill in 2003. He and the rest of the faculty members of Hispanic Studies have always challenged me to offer my best, and I consider myself fortunate to work with them in such a stimulating academic environment. Finally, this book would not exist without the constant support and understanding of my parents, my children, and especially my wife. If there is anything of value to be found in it, it is dedicated to them.

JOSÉ R. JOUVE MARTÍN
Montreal, September 2013

~

Introduction

In spite of their legal and racial status in colonial society, individuals of African descent, broadly referred in the documentation as *negros*, *mulatos*, and *pardos*, played a prominent role in the practice of medicine in Lima during the transition from the colonial to the republican period. Writing in the mid-nineteenth century, Peruvian satiric writer and journalist Manuel Atanasio Fuentes, who was a professor of legal medicine at the Universidad de San Marcos, called attention to this fact in his book *Lima: Apuntes históricos, descriptivos, estadísticos y de costumbres* (1866).[1] He praised the scientific education of the physicians of his age, whom he considered as competent as "those of other countries where there are good ones." As Fuentes makes clear, Peruvian medicine had not been so well regarded just eighty years earlier, when all that was necessary to "be received among the disciples of Galen" was "to have the inclination and to be black." To the best of his memory, "leaving aside the very respectable physicians Unanue, Tafur, Heredia, Paredes, and two or three more whites, the rest were not whiter than cinnamon." Despite this, he warned his readers to avoid drawing hasty conclusions regarding the quality of Peruvian medicine purely on the basis of race. Progress in the field certainly lagged far behind gains made in other sciences, but one should not assume that life in Lima at the turn of the nineteenth century was left in the hands of "ignorant and ludicrous quacks" (Fuentes 1985 [1867], 167). This was not the case. Many of those "quacks" were "individuals of talent who, thanks to their continuous studies, rose to the height of their profession in a country then so isolated from Europe. Doctors such as Valdés, Dávila, and Faustos, among others, were dark-skinned, but they were also able to make a name for themselves as learned and accredited physicians. Dr Montero, usually called *Doctor Santitos*, as black as any black man can be, was born with a gift for surgery" (ibid., 170).

Atanasio Fuentes was not the only observer to note the significant number of individuals of African origin active in Peruvian medicine. Archibald Smith, a British doctor who lived in Lima in the years following independence, wrote in his book *Peru as It Is* (1839) that, aside from a few physicians of European birth or descent, the majority of medical professionals "were raised from among the genuine black, or other more or less crossed Ethiopian castes, to whom, as is affirmed by Ayanque at page 43 of his celebrated satire, titled *Lima por dentro y fuera*, the healing art in all its branches, and especially surgery, was almost entirely entrusted" (Smith 1839, 1: 179).[2] According to Smith, the preponderance of these "Ethiopian castes" during the late colonial period arose from inadequate ideas entertained by the Spaniards, who viewed medicine "less as a noble science than as a superior sort of handicraft" (ibid., 1: 179–80). Another European, the Swiss naturalist Johan Jakob von Tschudi, who visited Peru in the late 1830s, also observed that most of the physicians in Lima were mulattoes (Von Tschudi 1854, 83). Contrary to Fuentes, however, he considered them to be "remarkable only for their ignorance, as they receive neither theoretical nor clinical instruction," despite which "they enjoy the full confidence of the public, who rank the ignorant native far above the educated foreigner" (ibid.). Peruvian authorities were not oblivious to the situation, nor were they particularly pleased with it. In the mid-eighteenth century, the viceroy even tried to ban Afro-Peruvians from the Faculty of Medicine at the University of San Marcos. Nevertheless, efforts at exclusion achieved only mixed results. According to Woodham, the strong presence of African descendants in the Peruvian medical field continued to be felt several decades after the implementation of those restrictions. Even Hipólito Unanue – Peru's foremost physician and intellectual figure in the late eighteenth and early nineteenth century – had to confront the common prejudice that characterized medicine as "an illiberal profession dominated by unschooled negroes and mulattoes" (1970, 124). In fact, Woodham remarks that Unanue's "own professors in the University of San Marcos de Lima, Gabriel

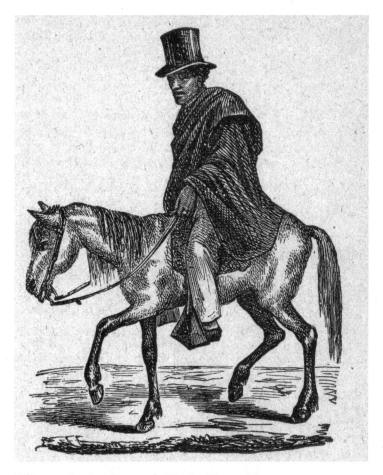

"El Doctor Santitos en su mula." Dr José Santos Montero was a surgeon active in the city hospitals of San Bartolomé and San Andrés.

Moreno and Cosme Bueno, were the only 'lights' in Peruvian medicine when Unanue arrived, and together they had held that honour for about twenty-five years" (ibid.).

Unfortunately, specific and detailed information about the activities of Afro-Peruvian surgeons and doctors is scarce, despite their apparent ubiquity. Contemporaries usually referred to them only in passing, without giving much information about their origins, contributions, or activities. For these reasons this book concentrates mainly on three particular medical practitioners. The first is José Manuel Valdés (1767–1843), an Afro-Peruvian categorized alternatively as *mulato* and *pardo*, who rose to the top medical position in Peru during the 1830s – that of Protomédico general de la República – after a distinguished career that began in the late 1780s. Valdés was the only person of African ancestry to have risen to a position of such scientific and political preeminence in nineteenth-century Spanish America. The second important figure in this book is José Manuel Dávalos (1758–1821). A *mulato*, born to a relatively affluent family, Dávalos was able to circumvent the legislation that prohibited persons of African origin from becoming doctors in Lima by studying in France. He obtained his doctorate from the University of Montpellier with a dissertation entitled *De morbis nonnullis Limae grassantibus ipsorumque therepeia* [On some common illnesses in Lima and their therapy] (1787). Together with Pedro Belomo, a doctor of Spanish descent, Dávalos took charge of the most important public health project in late colonial Peru: the smallpox vaccination campaigns. The third, and last, protagonist of this book, José Pastor de Larrinaga (1758–ca.1821), was one of the most famous – and controversial – surgeons of his era. He did not obtain the same level of social recognition as Valdés and Dávalos, and he was eventually publicly disgraced and discredited. Among his contemporaries, he was, nevertheless, the most vocal defender of the intellectual capacity and competence of Afro-Peruvians in the practice of surgery and medicine. Alongside these main figures, there were others whose names are mentioned in the sources, such as the doctor José María Dávila and the surgeons Mariano Faustos, José Puente, José Santos Montero, and Jerónimo de Utrilla. Unfortunately, information about their professional careers is extraordinarily limited because of the fragmented state of the archival record and the fact that, in contrast to Dávalos, Valdés, and Larrinaga, they did not leave any scientific writings behind.

The lives of Valdés, Dávalos, and Larrinaga radically question many existing assumptions about the relationship between race and knowledge in the cities of colonial and early republican Spanish America. The descendants of black slaves were not expected to be knowledgeable about – and even less to write on – the works of Hippocrates, Galen, or Sydenham. They were not supposed to comment from a scientific perspective on the causes of uterine cancer or dysentery, or to recommend the use of "fixed air" or special surgical instruments to alleviate a variety of painful physical conditions. They were not to be considered candidates for academic positions or given responsibility concerning health policy. And yet in Lima they did so. They actively joined the reform efforts of influential figures of the Peruvian Enlightenment such as Cosme Bueno and Hipólito Unanue. They became part of the scientific revolution that overtook the medical profession in Peru in the second half of the eighteenth century. They championed the theories of Herman Boerhaave and the School of Leyden and advocated for an empirical understanding of medicine that stressed the importance of the study of anatomy. It is true that their discussions did not bring about paradigmatic shifts, but they saw their work as an ongoing fight against superstition in a city where the curative powers of folk healers were frequently considered to exceed by far those of the most erudite doctors. As such, they proudly considered themselves as part of a modernization effort that would necessarily lead to the social and economic progress of the viceroyalty.

By the beginning of the nineteenth century, their success in the scientific world of Lima had given them a degree of authority that allowed them to address contemporary social, political, and philosophical issues. Their works touched in passing on Cornelius de Pauw's opinions on America, the need for burial reform in the Peruvian capital, the improvement in the field of midwifery, and the music and dances of African slaves, among other topics. This enabled them to present themselves not as simple medical practitioners but as *letrados* – members of the select group of writers and intellectuals that dominated the Peruvian world of letters. This fact is nicely captured in a speech given by Dávalos in 1798 as a candidate for the position of chair of Método de Medicina at the Universidad de San Marcos. After a lengthy exposition of the merits of his candidacy, Dávalos concluded that "from these [merits] it results that I am a qualified professor in each of the fields that are validated by this *Protomedicato* [chief medical office]: anatomy, chemistry, botany, natural philosophy, experimental physics, and more than competent in pure and mixed mathematics; but above all I am a public writer of substantial import" (1810, 17). Valdés and Larrinaga thought of themselves in much the same way.

To be sure, they saw science and writing not just as a medium through which to convey their ideas but also as part of a process of self-fashioning and differentiation that allowed them to distance themselves from other "darker" and less cultivated Afro-Peruvians. As scholars such as Bowser (1974), Blanchard (1992), Aguirre (1993), Hünefeldt (1994), and McKinley (2010; 2012) have noted, Lima's black community was far from a unified entity. It was fractured along legal (free men and slaves), ethnic (Bram, Bakongo, Wolof, etc.), racial (*negro, mulato, zambo, pardo*), professional (servants, artisans, professionals), and even gender lines (women made up a larger proportion of those who were free and had access to property). These "fracture lines" allowed for a wide variety of identities within the black community, which in turn helps explain the apparent paradox of individuals of African origin being themselves small slave owners. This multiplicity of identity positions prevented Lima's black community as a whole from becoming a unified political entity while allowing for the creation of smaller interest groups. In this regard, Valdés, Dávalos, and Larrinaga stressed that they were free *pardos* (individuals of African descent considered to be whiter than *mulatos*, both genealogically and racially, and therefore closer to Spaniards). As such they were especially interested in advancing the social status of those who shared their racial, legal, and professional identity. To a certain extent, theirs is a story of liberation, for they were able to break multiple racial and intellectual barriers, but they were far from being revolutionaries. They may have advocated a more humane treatment for black slaves and other *negros*, but even acknowledging that they shared in part the same origins, they did not consider them their equals. Of the three, only Larrinaga adopted a more inclusive stance with regard to the right to knowledge and freedom of all Afro-Peruvians.

From a chronological point of view, the bulk of this book concentrates on an eighty-year period (1760–1840) during which the medical careers of Valdés, Dávalos, and Larrinaga were developing and Peru was transforming from a colony to an independent state. The history of black medical practitioners in Peru, however, dates back to a much earlier time. Black healers began to emerge in the mid-sixteenth century, when the first African slaves arrived in Peru and intermingled with the growing number of Iberian and indigenous *curanderos* (folk healers). Accordingly, the first chapter of this book, "From Healers to Doctors," provides a historical introduction to the participation of *negros* and *mulatos* in Peruvian medicine, from Lima's founding in 1535 until 1791, when José Pastor de Larrinaga published a passionate defence of black surgeons entitled *Apología de los cirujanos del Perú*. In this chapter, I argue that the presence of individuals of African descent in the medical profession can be attributed to a combination of factors: the racial demographics of the capital of the viceroyalty; the chronic lack of qualified doctors and surgeons; the frequently contradictory stance that Spanish authorities took concerning the participation of blacks in higher education; and the relative flexibility of the caste system in colonial Lima. However, while their medical abilities were generally held in high esteem, the special place that Valdés, Dávalos, and Larrinaga occupied in Peruvian medicine cannot be understood without taking into account their relationship with Hipólito Unanue and his plans to reform Peruvian medicine. It was he who really opened the (predominantly white) intellectual world of Lima to them.

Chapter 2, "Enlightened Surgeons, Public Writers," explores how these surgeons and doctors expressed their medical and social ideas in the public sphere. While Dávalos published his dissertation in Montpellier, Unanue gave Valdés and Larrianga the chance of finding their own intellectual space in the *Mercurio peruano*, one of the most important venues for the dissemination of the scientific revolution in South America. They took the opportunity to defend the value of surgery for the advancement of medicine and to comment on the politics of reproduction and demographic growth, a topic that was at the centre of Unanue's reformist agenda. Their articles aimed as much at advancing knowledge as enlightening a society which they considered plagued by unsound medical practices. Some of the articles – especially those submitted by Larrinaga – proved controversial and were hotly disputed by other contributors to the *Mercurio peruano*. Nevertheless, they exemplified the new scientific status accorded to surgery and surgeons in late colonial society and the important role given to those who were on the front lines of medical care in Peru. The *Mercurio peruano* also allowed them to develop their status as *letrados*, able to write not only about surgical procedures but also about philosophy, theology, and history.

In Chapter 3, "Doctors, Citizens, Revolutionaries," I discuss the rise of Valdés and Dávalos as two of Lima's most influential doctors, and

Larrinaga's fall in disgrace as a result of his public confrontation with Hipólito Unanue in the first decade of the nineteenth century. The attention of this group of physicians shifted from science to politics as the French invasion of Spain and the convocation of the Cortes de Cádiz created in Lima the conditions for an open discussion of the citizenship rights of individuals of African descent. This was a cause which the *pardos* of Lima enthusiastically supported, but in their politics, as in their scientific opinions, Valdés, Dávalos, and Larrinaga were more divided than it seemed. Once absolutist rule was restored in 1814, Larrinaga made it clear that his loyalties lay with Ferdinand VII, a position that owed much to his ongoing confrontation with Unanue. For their part, Valdés and Dávalos sided with doctors who – like Unanue – pragmatically accepted the monarchy's return. But even if they paid lip service to colonial authorities, there is little doubt about the nature of their political leanings. Both Dávalos and Valdés greeted Peru's independence with joy. In fact, Dávalos was among those who signed Peru's declaration of independence (Pamo Reina 2009, 63; Odriozola 1877, 39). For his part, Valdés went on to write an ode to the Argentine general José de San Martín, celebrating the liberation of Lima in 1821, and to Simón Bolívar in 1824 upon his appointment by the Peruvian congress as dictator of Peru.

Chapter 4, "A Black Protomédico in Republican Peru," tells the story of José Manuel Valdés's ascent to the apex of the medical profession in Peru. Valdés acted first as the aide-de-camp to the *protomédico* (chief medical officer) Miguel Tafur and was later promoted to *Protomédico general de la República* (chief medical officer of the Republic). In that position, he assumed the task of creating a "national" medicine based on three objectives: (1) reasserting the authority of the chief medical office, the Protomedicato, over the practice of medicine in the volatile political context of republican Peru; (2) developing Peruvian medicine so that it could rise to prominence in the burgeoning and somewhat chauvinistic world of modern science; and (3) defending the intellectual and economic interests of Peruvian doctors *vis-à-vis* their foreign counterparts. These three goals were hotly contested. The authority of the Protomedicato was challenged by a combination of folk healers and political liberals, who would recognize neither Tafur's nor Valdés's authority and defended the idea that medicine should be an open market, free from "tyrannical" restrictions. For its part, the project of creating a "national" and "independent" medicine that could rival established European medical traditions was questioned by those who emerged as the neocolonial guardians of scientific orthodoxy in independent Peru – namely, the British physicians. Finally, while many Peruvian doctors approved of Valdés's actions in support of their economic interests, a growing number of them resented the complete supervision of their medical practice that Valdés sought to impose as a trade-off for his protectionism.

In the concluding section of this book, I use Valdés's reinterpretation of the life of a seventeenth-century mulatto surgeon, Brother Martín de Porres, to reflect on the ways in which, for a time, the descendants of slaves in Peru became healers, surgeons, and doctors. Valdés saw in the friar Martín de Porres not only a physician and a "miracle maker" but also a moral model for the new republic and for those who shared similar racial origins. Nevertheless, Valdés was far from being a radical libertarian. While he strived throughout his life to increase the participation of the *castas* in the public sphere, he opted to remain silent about the more contentious issue of African slavery. Valdés's death in 1843 marked the end of the participation of individuals of African descent in Peruvian medicine and surgery. The demographic changes of the city of Lima, together with the rising social prestige of surgery as a medical discipline, meant that even though slavery and caste legislation had been abolished, blacks and mulattoes no longer had the opportunitiy to become part of the medical profession. Paradoxically, Valdés's rise to the position of Protomédico general de la República, his crowning achievement, also represented the end of the tradition of black medical practitioners that had started three centuries earlier.

The chapters of this book are an exploration of both the black experience and the politics of medicine in colonial Peru. While African healing practices in the Americas have received significant attention (Laguerre 1988; Voeks 1993; Weaver 2006; Garofalo 2006; Sweet 2011), works on black doctors and surgeons remain scarce, despite a wealth of archival evidence that suggests that their presence was more significant than previously thought (Vidal Ortega 2002, 271; Goodwin 2009, 38; Hinton 2004, 11; Lanning 1985, 87–91; Mott 2005, 41). In this regard, Lima offers a case that allows us to look not only at the medical beliefs of these practitioners but also at the role they played in the dissemination of the scientific revolution and in shaping the sanitary life of the city, both on the front lines of medical care and in the administration of public policy. Given their relevance, it is surprising that few studies have been devoted to this group of black physicians and their relationship with the main figures of the Peruvian Enlightenment. The studies that do exist have been published only in Peru, and they enjoyed limited circulation or are already out of print (Paz Soldán 1942; López Martínez 1993; Rabí Chara 2006b). A notable exception is that of Warren (2010), whose book on colonial medicine in Peru documents some of their activities while focusing on the debates about medical reform and population growth.

In order to practise their trade and find a space in the scientific world of colonial Lima, Valdés, Larrinaga, and Dávalos did not have to forge any documents to pass as whites, nor did they use legal means to "cleanse" their "blood," such as the famous *gracias al sacar* certificates issued by the late colonial administration (Twinam 2009). While racial identities during this period were more fluid than previously accepted – as evidenced by a growing body of secondary literature (Castleman 2001; Carrera 2003; Barvosa 2008; Fisher and O'Hara 2009; Rappaport, forthcoming) – they did not have to renounce their *casta* to achieve their goals. On the contrary, they were openly classified as *mulatos* or *pardos* by their contemporaries, and they identified themselves as such. In spite of this, they assigned much more importance to their professional identity than to their racial one, and so did others. They were accepted by Hipólito Unanue and other white physicians because of their academic knowledge and professional abilities and not out of sympathy for their plight as members of a disadvantaged social group. Once established, professional identities – particularly in the liberal professions – sometimes played a stronger role than race in assigning the social status of an individual in colonial Lima, at least for the most progressive sector of the colonial elite. Unsurprisingly, most of their writings do not mention their race at all, and neither did their interlocutors. They simply identified themselves as surgeons, doctors, or writers and expected to be treated as such.

This does not mean that race was unimportant. On the contrary, Lima's medical world was extraordinarily hierarchical. Phlebotomists, Romance surgeons, Latin surgeons, doctors, and university professors formed a pyramid, at the peak of which was the colony's protomédico. Others at the top (doctors and university professors) were predominantly white; those at the bottom (phlebotomists, Romance surgeons, and Latin surgeons) were *negros*, *mulatos*, or *mestizos*. Professional disputes – as there were between surgeons and doctors about the boundaries of their respective professions – frequently concealed racial fears and apprehensions. Moreover, not all white physicians and colonial bureaucrats were as open-minded as the group led by Unanue. Some of them sought to and, for a time, succeeded in blocking the access of people of African descent to the medical profession. In fact, the attempts made by some European surgeons to prohibit men of African descent from practising surgery in Lima was the impetus for Larrinaga to write his *Apología de los cirujanos del Perú* in the 1790s.

Apart from contributing to the advancement of science, the practice of medicine also offered Afro-Peruvians a platform from which to defend their political rights and participate in the process of nation building, a topic that has attracted increasing attention (Naro 2003; Knight 2003; Blanchard 2008; Andrews 2004, 11–116; 2010). As I discuss in chapter 3 of this book, the French invasion of Spain and the drafting of the Cadiz Constitution of 1812 opened the door for the debates on the citizenship rights of those of African origin. This was a subject closely followed by the black elite of Lima, many of whose members were surgeons or doctors who highlighted their many contributions to the progress of medicine and the health of their fellow citizens. After independence, Valdés's role at the Protomédicato general de la República and his rise to the position of protomédico allowed him to shape the health policy of the new nation and develop his vision of Peruvian medicine. The zeal that he demonstrated in this task inspired his enemies to award him the unflattering title of Medical Dictator of Peru. In this regard, this book is a contribution to the ongoing research on the history of the black presence in Peru, and it seeks to expand the studies carried out by Aguirre (1993), Hünefeldt (1994), and Blanchard (1992), among others, by looking at this community from an angle that takes science rather than slavery as the focal point.

Even though most of the black doctors discussed in this book never left Peru, their experiences have broader implications for our understanding of the interrelation of science, medicine, and the black experience in the Atlantic world. One of them who did traverse the Atlantic was José Manuel Dávalos, who left Lima to study in Montpellier to circumvent the colonial legislation that restricted mulattoes from becoming doctors. His dissertation, published in 1787, was well received in both France and Spain. The journal *Espíritu de los mejores diarios literarios que se publican en Europa*, a publication that collected news published in other European languages for a Spanish readership, observed that Dávalos's work had been favourably reviewed by the *Journal encyclopédique* in France, which considered that his book announced "the arrival of a true talent with great intellectual penetration, profound erudition, sound critical judgment, substantiated opinions, enlightened practice, and a gift for observation" (1787, 599). Unlike the case of Domingo Álvares studied by Sweet (2011), Dávalos returned to Lima not as an African healer but as a full-fledged doctor graduated from one of Europe's most prestigious faculties of medicine. His standing among his colleagues was due in no small part to this fact. For those black physicians who remained in Lima, contact with the medical and healing traditions of the Atlantic world took many forms. For instance, the European surgeons and doctors who arrived periodically in the city aboard navy and merchant ships frequently offered opportunities for the exchange of ideas, but these exchanges also caused friction. As Salvany and others soon learned, Lima's medical community was fiercely independent and did not take foreign criticism lightly. This does not mean that it was ignorant of European medical developments. On the contrary, physicians such as Valdés, Dávalos, and Larrinaga frequently referenced the most important medical writers of their age in their work. Their writings illustrate something that historians have amply noted throughout the past decade, namely that in spite of the distance that separated Peru from the main scientific societies of the Old Continent, the Spanish colonies were not oblivious to the advances made during the Enlightenment and the scientific revolution (Warren 2010; Cañizares-Esguerra 2006; Barrera-Osorio 2006).

Scholars who have tried to reconstruct the intellectual history of African slaves and their descendants in colonial Latin America are fully aware of the extreme difficulty of doing so on account of the scarcity of surviving texts. The fact that the stories of José Manuel Valdés, José Manuel Dávalos, and José Pastor Larrinaga can be retold at all is extraordinary, and even more so because we can use their own words. This book seeks to restore their writing and voices to their rightful place. In doing so, it joins the efforts of Jackson (1997), Luis (2007), Van Deusen (2004), Nwankwo (2005), and Acree and Borucki (2010), among others. The texts of these black physicians are not, however, an expression of "blackness" in a postcolonial sense. Stylistically, their texts were virtually indistinguishable from the work of their white peers. Moreover, some of the examples they employed to illustrate their medical ideas and theories intentionally emphasized the distance between them and the general Afro-Peruvian population, and they did not hesitate to criticize what they saw as the barbarous customs and superstitions of African slaves. Yet their writings are very significant. They clearly demonstrate that those who belonged to the "Ethiopian castes," as Archibald Smith called them, were able to interact with colonial written culture in a more extensive way than previously acknowledged and in a wider variety of settings than usually assumed (Jouve Martín 2005). Valdés, Dávalos, and Larrinaga considered themselves not just medical professionals but writers, and they wrote not only scientific essays but also poetry, biographies, and even religious works. Undoubtedly, Unanue played a critical role in "empowering" these black intellectuals, and for the most part they played by his rules, but as the case of Larrinaga illustrates, they were also able to challenge his authority, albeit at a hefty professional and economic cost.

Valdés, Dávalos, and Larrinaga left behind a substantial body of written work that appeared in different venues. Even though Lima was the most frequent place of publication for their writings, some were published in places far removed from Peru: Dávalos's doctoral dissertation appeared in Montpellier; Larrinaga's *Apología de los cirujanos del Perú* was published in Granada under the auspices of his patron, Archbishop Juan Manuel Moscoso y Peralta, a former Bishop of Cuzco; and Valdés's collection of essays, *Disertaciones médico-quirúrgicas sobre varios puntos importantes* (1815), was printed in Madrid. This illustrates the fact that they went to great lengths to ensure the dissemination of their ideas and considered them to be relevant beyond the borders of Peru. As a result, many of their works are scattered in different national and university libraries in Peru, Spain, and the United States. Valdés, Dávalos, and Larrinaga also contributed to scientific and political journals edited in Lima, such as the *Mercurio peruano*, and collaborated on pamphlets that were produced by the popular press of J. Masías. After independence, Valdés became particularly active in newspapers such as *El Regenerador* and *El Comercio*, which are currently stored in the Biblioteca nacional del Perú as well as in the

archives of the Instituto Riva-Agüero in Lima. Archival documents used
to support the findings of this research come from the Archivo general
de la Nación (Lima), Archivo de Indias (Madrid), and Archivo histórico
nacional (Madrid), among others.

Before I conclude, I would like to offer a brief commentary about
the use of racial terminology in this monograph. Throughout the book,
I use various racial terms in both English and Spanish to refer to individuals of African ancestry living in Peru prior to the mid-nineteenth
century. Inevitably, modern and historical uses of the terms overlap.
Translating Spanish colonial racial terminology into English presents
the well-known problem that racial categorization systems were substantially different in Spanish colonial America and North America,
even when they used similar words (Wade 1997; Thomson 2011;
O'Toole 2012). I normally use the terms "black" and "Afro-Peruvian"
as synonymous in reference to those who were of African ancestry,
independently of whether they were further classified as "blacks" or
negros (Africans and their descendants who had undergone no racial
mixing), as *mulatos* (mixed Spanish and African ancestry), as *zambos*
(mixed indigenous and African ancestry) or any other of the multitude
of racial terms reflected in colonial documents (Carrera 2003; Katzew
2004; Deans-Smith 2005). I think that the context makes it clear in
all instances when I am using "black" or "negro" as a general designation and when I am using those words to refer to the *casta* of a
specific individual or group of individuals. Nevertheless, one must take
into account that, despite the orderly world created by *casta* paintings,
the use of racial designations in colonial Spanish America was far from
an exact science. The documentation offers multiple instances in which
the same individual is classified variously as *negro* and as *mulato*
depending on the different scribes in charge of writing the document
and occasionally even when the scribe was the same person. In this
sense, ambiguity is frequently embedded in the sources themselves. The
term *pardo* designates an individual of especially fair complexion, but
it was not significantly different from *mulato* from a legal perspective.
Mulatos and *pardos* tried their best to differentiate themselves from
negros as a way to improve their standing in colonial society, but they
were only partially successful. Although colonial legislation and social
custom were sometimes more lenient with mulattoes than with those
of pure African ancestry, colonial officials frequently grouped *negros*

and *mulatos* together as being part of the same group, disregarding their differences. This was something that Valdés, who was widely seen as a *mulato* or *pardo*, learned the hard way in 1815. After having earned almost universal praise in Lima for his medical career, he had to give up his aspiration to become a member of the church because of the indignation it produced in the *cabildo catedralicio* (cathedral's council), some of whose members complained that "they would soon have to share their seats in the cathedral chorus with a *negro*" (Lavalle n.d., 11). According to Lavalle, Valdés concluded that it "must not be God's will that he should become a priest and that the opposition from the ecclesiastical council was a merited punishment for his pride" (ibid.). No matter how far from Africa *pardos* and *mulatos* considered their roots to be, colonial authorities saw fit to curb their ambitions by reminding them from time to time what they considered their true origins.

THE
BLACK
DOCTORS
OF
COLONIAL LIMA

CHAPTER 1

From Healers to Doctors

At the end of the eighteenth century, Lima had become a complex multiracial society. Writing in 1681, the Dominican priest Juan Meléndez could still argue in his *Tesoros verdaderos de las Indias* that in Peru there were just three "nations" (*indios*, *negros*, and *españoles*). Members of each nation rarely "married outside their group," most marriages being "of *indios* with *indios*, *españoles* with *españoles*, and *negros* with *negros*." According to Meléndez, *indios* and *españoles* tried particularly hard not to mix in marriage with people from a different caste "because they want their blood to run pure and without mixture in all their progeny." Based on that assertion, Mélendez could even claim that in Peru "the *indio* is and has always been *indio*, the *español* is and has always been *español*, and the *negro* is and has always been *negro*" (Meléndez 1681, 352). If it was difficult to uphold Meléndez's claims in late-seventeenth-century Lima – the historical record and most other accounts offer exactly the opposite view – it became impossible to do so by the mid-eighteenth century, in spite of the Herculean efforts made by the church and the colonial administration to discourage racial mixing (McKinley 2010). Viceroy José Antonio de Velasco, Count of Superunda, attested to the alleged chaos caused by the preponderance of the *castas* in mid-eighteenth-century Lima when he wrote to the Crown:

> There are [in the city] many *mestizos*, *negros*, and *mulatos* as well as individuals of other *castas*, but their number is impossible to ascertain, and when we have tried to determine it, they

have suspected that we wanted to impose more taxes and force labour on them ... There are very few people in this kingdom with white skin who can be distinguished by the name of *españoles*, and their number does not grow despite the large influx of persons that come here from Spain due to the poor fecundity of [white] women and the weak complexion of their offspring, and there are many who, with reason, complain that their sons cannot have an appropriate secular career and are forced to become part of the Church. *(Memorias de los virreyes* 1859, 79)

Colonial legislation succeeded in establishing a racial order that clearly privileged the white elite, but as the Count of Superunda made clear in his report, it had failed in its attempt to limit access to "secular careers" to those of European origin only. Blacks, mulattoes, and other *castas* of African descent were able to make a living as artisans and members of the various guilds. Others were able to fill positions in the colonial bureaucracy, as illustrated by the Royal Decree of 1621, which denounced the fact that several of them had become public notaries in Lima (Konetzke 1958, 2.1: 260). Some even became legitimate members of the church, as illustrated by the ordination of a mulatto named Francisco de Santa Fe as a priest in 1663 (AAL, Orden de Predicadores de Santo Domingo, file III, dossier 13, 18 fs; for more on mulattoes and the religious orders, see van Deusen 2004). In fact, the city demographics and the white elite's disregard for certain professions made it almost inevitable to admit some *negros* and *mulatos* into "secular careers" in order to ensure that basic necessary services remained staffed. As we shall see in this chapter, this was particularly the case of medicine and more specifically surgery, which rapidly became a multiracial profession. To see how this happened, we will start by looking at the situation at the end of the eighteenth century through the lens of the mulatto surgeon José Pastor de Larrinaga.

A Surgeon's Defence

Born in 1758 into a family of modest economic means but strong social connections, José Pastor de Larrinaga was the legitimate son of Pedro José de Larrinaga, a white man, and Gregoria Hurtado, a black woman. Larrinaga's mother was the *hermana de leche*[1] of Catalina

Hurtado y Peralta, a Spanish noblewoman who was the cousin of Juan Manuel Moscoso y Peralta, bishop of Cuzco and later archbishop of Granada (Rabi Chara 2006b, 21).[2] Godfathered by members of her influential family, the young Larrinaga soon found himself studying at the school of San Francisco de Jesús in Lima. After graduation, he joined the Hospital de San Bartolomé, where he began practising as a medical assistant under the supervision of Tomás Obregón, the hospital's *enfermero mayor,* or chief nurse (ibid., 21–2). Larrinaga successfully passed the exam to become a Latin surgeon in 1778, and in 1780 he became a military surgeon in the Regimiento de Milicias de Dragones de Caraballo, a cavalry unit. He held that position until 1807, when he was replaced by Pedro Utrilla – a descendant of the Utrilla family mentioned by Valle y Caviedes in *Diente del Parnaso* – following a bitter professional and legal dispute (ibid., 205–6). In addition to working as a surgeon for several hospitals and city monasteries, he soon found himself at the service and under the protection of the house of Bishop Juan Manuel Moscoso y Peralta, whom he regarded as "the protector of the sciences and of all of those who have cultivated them in this Hemisphere" (Larrinaga 1791, ii).

As their correspondence attests, Larrinaga was able to keep the lines of communication open with Moscoso y Peralta even after he had left Peru for the Archbishopric of Granada in 1789. These endeavours culminated with the archbishop's patronage of Larrinaga's first work, *Apología de los Cirujanos del Perú*, which was published at Moscoso y Peralta's expense in Granada – albeit with a modest print run of 400 copies – and shipped to Larrinaga for distribution in Lima (Rabi Chara 2006b, 18). Larrinaga's aim in writing the book was threefold: first, to legitimate the right of individuals of African descent to practise the profession of surgery in spite of their African origins; secondly, to denounce the unfair meddling of *cirujanos ultramarinos* (overseas surgeons) in the city's medical affairs; and finally, to disprove the thesis of Dutch geographer and philosopher Cornelius de Pauw with regard to the inhabitants of America and the state of academic learning in Peru.

The overseas surgeons who Larrinaga found so contemptuous were those who arrived periodically on the coasts of Lima onboard merchant and naval ships. Their number and presence had greatly increased in the second half of the eighteenth century following a series of reforms introduced by the Spanish navy. While fully trained surgeons were rarely found as part of a ship's crew in the sixteenth and seventeenth centuries, this situation changed through the recognition that proper medical care was a key element in the modernization of the royal fleet.[3] The medical modernization of the Spanish navy was accomplished through the creation of the position of Cirujano mayor de la Armada in 1708, and later through the foundation of the Real Colegio de cirugía de Cádiz in 1748. As a result, surgeons educated by and for the Spanish navy were among the most capable surgeons in the entire Spanish empire (Aragón Espeso 2009, 117–31). As proud graduates of the Real Colegio de cirugía de Cádiz and similar institutions, naval surgeons frequently found themselves at odds with their colonial counterparts, whose knowledge and abilities they considered inferior. The situation was made worse by the fact that naval surgeons and physicians were authorized to practise their trade not only on board ships and in navy hospitals but also in the private houses where their patients recovered (Ordenanzas 1974 [1678], f. 30). As if that was not enough, naval surgeons were also encouraged to meet with "the professors of renowned hospitals in the ports where they arrived" (Ordenanzas generales de la Armada naval 1793, 382–3).

In a city such as Lima, where many of those who practised surgery were reputedly of African descent, conflict seemed inevitable. Disputes between Peninsular and Peruvian surgeons soon erupted, centring not only on technical issues but also more broadly on the racial origins and presumed intellectual inferiority of those born in America. In fact, the incident that led to the publication of Larrinaga's essay had arisen some months earlier, when a group of these overseas physicians tried to block the employment of a mulatto surgeon who, "full of practical knowledge and with more than thirty years of service and merits," had been hired by the Real hospital de Santa Ana. The cirujanos ultramarinos had argued that the surgeon should not have been given the job, since "mulattoes should not practise surgery in the royal hospitals of the city of Lima" (Larrinaga 1791, 2). They supported their pretension "with the authority and weight of the royal decree issued by King Ferdinand VI on 27 September 1752, which ordered the provost of the Universidad de San Marcos to forbid the registration and graduation of those who were not legitimately classified as españoles" (ibid., 17). Ferdinand VI's decree did indeed prevent mulattoes from obtaining academic degrees from the Universidad de San Marcos and asked colonial authorities to void the titles that had already been granted. In spite of this, it did not expressly forbid people of African origin from practising as surgeons in the city hospitals, for which all they needed was a certificate from the Protomedicato and not a university degree. Thus, for Larrinaga the issue was simple: "If they were only to read that decree and were made aware that a hospital is one thing and a university is another ... everything would be solved" (ibid.).

Prominent among those who provided overseas surgeons with ideological ammunition for their views was Dutch philosospher and geographer Cornelius de Pauw. A vocal critic of the racial origins of Americans, he had already denounced Peruvian institutions of higher education in his highly influential *Recherches philosophiques sur les Américains* (1770). For him, "the universities in the Americas have not produced any notable creole men. Not a single one of those who have graduated from the university of San Marcos in Lima has ever been able to write even a bad book despite the fame of this institution compared with other universities in the Americas"; American institutions had repeatedly proved their inability to produce "any grand master, philosopher, doctor, physicist, or intellectual whose name could cross the sea and be appreciated in Europe" (Pauw 1770, 2: 166–7). This lack of *hommes célèbres* could not be attributed simply to "the general ignorance, the professors' barbarism, or the deplorable state to which the sciences have been reduced in the Indies"; rather, it was because of the vices and temperament of the inhabitants of that region (ibid., 2: 167). Following Buffon, de Pauw argued that the imperfect character and physical constitution of the Indians and of those born in America was due primarily to geography and climate as well as to the perverse effects of the mixture of races (ibid., 1: 40).[4]

Like other colonial intellectuals both inside and outside Peru (Gerbi 2010, 289–324), Larrinaga had no patience for those who propagated such defamatory views. He argued that Peruvian authors had printed their works in both Lima and Madrid since the seventeenth century. He added that if there appeared to be a scarcity of Peruvian books, it was because the expense associated with the publication of such works "has suffocated in darkness and oblivion many manuscripts that the *literatti* of this city keep with even more care than if they were in print" (Larrinaga 1791, x–xi). In this regard, Larrinaga pointed out that "in Lima, a manuscript is more costly than six books printed in Madrid ...

Thus, it is not surprising that there are so few public writers in a country that produces many substantial works, as other authors who know more than the intemperate de Pauw have noted" (ibid., x). In Larrinaga's opinion, de Pauw had mistakenly identified as an intellectual problem what was clearly an economic one. Despite this, Larrinaga's main criticism of de Pauw centred not on the economics of colonial publication but on the Dutch philosopher's affirmations concerning the supposed inferiority of those born in America in relation to the northern races.

"Whites born in the northern nations," countered Larrinaga, "are not necessarily more ingenious than those who are born in the southern regions" (1791, 2–3). Far from being limited to any specific country or continent, the arts and sciences were destined to flourish wherever there was "ingenuity, application, and good taste" (ibid., 4). Moreover, Larrinaga proudly noted that "the difference in the colour of one's skin does not affect the qualities of one's soul, and those of dark and olive-coloured skin alike enjoy the blessing of being wise if they have the necessary attributes to be so. Therefore, nobody should blame the accidental veneer with which nature has endowed men, since it's not the body but the soul that constitutes the spiritual and philosophical life that we enjoy" (ibid.). As for those who argued that slavery had left an indelible stain on mulatto surgeons, Larrinaga replied with indignation: "On what can they base the criticism of our creole surgeons whose fathers were blacks or slaves if we know that, in practice, the spirit cannot be captured, much less have colour?" (ibid., 6). He considered it a fundamental error to maintain that "because the fathers were slaves, the sons would not be able to embrace the natural sciences" – an argument that demanded its proponents to prove "with positive facts that one can shackle the spirit along with the hands" (ibid.).

Larrinaga proudly noted that at the time of his writing there were 56 surgeons in the city of Lima, most of whom were mulattoes, and that "in 256 years since the founding of the city there have been almost no surgeons other than mulattoes in the military expeditions and navy, in the hospitals, in the palaces and in the religious communities, etc." (ibid., 17–18).[5] Larrinaga reminded readers that Spanish law itself guaranteed their employment "as noted by Mr Solórzano in Book 2, Chapter 30, Articles 19, 20, and 21 of his *Política indiana*," according to which, "if these men [*mulatos* and *mestizos*] were born of a legitimate matrimony and do not fall victim to another vice or defect that would impede them, they can and should consider themselves citizens of the provinces of the Indies and be allowed access to the appropriate honours and offices" (ibid., 24).[6] But even if that were not the case, who would fill their positions, Larrinaga challenged his readers to explain, if mulattoes were to be forbidden from becoming surgeons or from practising their profession in the city hospitals: "Will young men from Europe come to Lima only to practise surgery? Of our Spanish Americans, will those having the talent to be doctors want to lower themselves to be practitioners of surgery? And then, who will occupy the positions of *barchilones, jeringuero, untador*, second nurse, and first nurse?" (ibid., 31).[7]

Larrinaga considered the answers to these questions to be obvious. No member of the white elite would ever be willing to fill these demanding and frequently underpaid positions, and he warned the viceregal authorities that they risked a health crisis if they prohibited mulatto surgeons from practising their trade (Warren 2010, 66). In fact, a defiant Larrinaga concluded that colonial society at large and the white elite in particular were "even more interested than we are in conserving and encouraging those who have worked for its benefit for 180 years" (Larrinaga 1791, 21).

Caring for a Black City

Founded by Francisco Pizarro on 18 January 1535, Lima was erected on the banks of the Rimac River, close to the Pacific Ocean and to what was then a small indigenous settlement. Early settlers were composed mainly of Spanish conquistadors, the original indigenous population, and the small retinue of African slaves that the Spaniards had brought with them (Lockhardt 1994, 193–224; Restall 2000, 171–205). They were attended by a small army of surgeons, barbers, and phlebotomists who practised various surgical and medical procedures for a modest fee (Lastres 1951a, 79). Many of them lacked proper academic and professional certification, which did not stop them from lobbying the city council for permission to practise medicine. They argued that their documents had been lost during the hardships of the conquest or mislaid in the long and perilous journey from the metropolis. Confronted with a shortage of properly educated doctors and with a rising population, the colonial authorities frequently had no other option than to grant them permission to practise (Lanning 1985, 45–6). Inevitably, the quality of medical care suffered and, as a result, complaints about the city's physicians and the price and poor quality of the medicines they prescribed did not take long to appear (*Libro primero de Cabildos de Lima*, 1888, 1: 169). This situation was compounded by the many folk healers, impostors, and tricksters who claimed to be able to cure all kinds of illnesses with remedies that many in Lima considered much better than those prescribed by the approved physicians. The colonial authorities' efforts to address the problem yielded only mixed results. Physicians and other medical practitioners in Spain had, since the fifteenth century, been under the authority of the Tribunal del Protomedicato.[8] Early attempts to establish the tribunal in Lima were, however, far from successful. The king appointed the first protomédico, Hernaldo de Sepúlveda, in 1537, but only two years after arriving in Peru, Sepúlveda petitioned the municipal council to allow him to leave Lima and return to Santo Domingo (*Libros de Cabildos de Lima* 1935, 1: 359). Thirty years passed before the next royal *protomédico*, Dr Antonio Sánchez Renedo, was welcomed to the viceroyalty. Sánchez Renedo was granted powers similar to those that protomédicos enjoyed in Spain, including the inspection and certification of physicians, surgeons, and apothecaries (Lanning 1985, 29). After his death in 1578, two local physicians, Álvaro de Otres and Fulano Henríquez, were appointed as interim protomédicos until the arrival of Íñigo de Hormero from Spain in 1589. It was only then that an era of relative stability in Lima's Tribunal del Protomedicato began. This fact, together with the establishment of the Faculty of Medicine at the University of San Marcos in 1634, helped regularize the practice of medicine in the capital of Peru.[9] Nevertheless, the definitive consolidation of academic and administrative power came only in 1646 when Phillip IV mandated that the professor of Prima de Medicina at San Marcos would, by definition, become head of the Protomedicato (ibid., 30; *Recopilación* libro 5, título 6, ley 3).

Medical care in Lima rapidly became racially and socially stratified, at least on paper. Hospitals targeted different social groups, which helped in turn to consolidate and reinforce racial divisions (Cahill 1995, 125). By 1538, the city had already established the future site of its first hospital, the Hospital Real de San Andrés de los Españoles, which became operational in 1550 (Barbagelata 1945, 56). It was initially devoted to the care of Spaniards of poor economic means who did not have access to medical care in their homes, but it eventually admitted blacks and individuals of mixed descent, albeit segregated in different rooms (Cahill 1995, 137–8). In 1549 Archbishop Gerónimo de Loayza founded the Hospital de Santa Ana de los Naturales, to provide medical and spiritual care to the indigenous population of the city so that Indians could not only be healed of their illnesses and wounds, but – as Bernabé Cobo recalled in his *Historia de la fundación de Lima* – so that they could also be "instructed in the matters of our Holy Catholic Faith and receive the Sacraments" (Cobo 1882 [1639], 307). According to an eighteenth-century reprint of the hospital's constitution, black patients were explicitly banned because of the damage and wrongs they had inflicted on the hospital and the Indians in the past (*Constituciones y ordenanzas del Hospital Real de Santa Ana*, 1778, art. 33). But even if patients were being racially separated, the individuals who took care of them generally were not, and the city hospitals had already become a racial melting pot by the end of the sixteenth century. The Indian patients in the Hospital de Santa Ana de los Naturales, for example, were cared for by three priests as well as "twenty-seven African slaves who worked as nurses, bookkeepers, cooks and laundresses," (van Deusen 1999, 9), in addition to a doctor, a surgeon, an apothecary, and a barber for whom no racial description was provided (Cobo 1882 [1639], 310; *Constituciones del Hospital Real de Santa Ana* 1778, art. 42–56).[10] Gender and socio-economic status also played an important role. Spanish women of limited economic means were cared for mostly at the Hospital de San Cosme and San Damián, also known as Hospital de la Caridad, located at the Plaza de la Inquisición. Half hospital, half convent, it also accepted *mestizas, mulatas*, and free black women, thereby blurring the racial distinctions among those who belonged to the most disadvantaged sectors of colonial society (Cobo 1882 [1639], 313).

The slave trade had a major impact on the sanitary infrastructure of the city. It had begun as a relatively modest business, but the discovery of the riches of Potosí and the political consolidation of the viceroyalty of Peru led to such a rapid increase in the demand for African slaves that by the end of the sixteenth century, the Peruvian capital had become a prominent market as well as a distribution centre for other parts of South America (Bowser 1974, 55). Slaves were brought to Lima and its environs to work on nearby *haciendas* and be employed as servants or temporary workers, most living in their master's home or in communal housing known as *callejones* (Higgins 2005, 77). The African presence in the city became even more visible with the decline of the indigenous population and its resettlement in the nearby town of Santiago del Cercado, which started in 1570 and ended in 1590 (Barbagelata 1945, 59). A head count carried out by Archbishop Toribio de Mogrovejo in 1593 estimated Lima's population at 12,790, of which almost half – 6,690 – were *negros* or *mulatos* (AGI, Patronato, 248, 28; Bowser 1974, 339). By 1614 the city's population had grown substantially, according to a census ordered by Viceroy Marquis de Montesclaros, but the ratio of European and African residents remained stubbornly stable: 12,000 Spaniards compared with 11,000 blacks and mulattoes, and just over 2,000 Indians and mestizos (Salinas y Córdova 1957 [1630], 245). Deeply worried about the massive presence of African slaves and freemen, the colonial authorities commissioned a new *numeración* only five years later, in 1619, which did nothing to alleviate their concerns. On the contrary, it revealed the striking fact that, for the first time, there were more African *castas* than Europeans in the city, having accounted for 11,997 blacks and 1,116 mulattoes, while only 9,706 individuals were classified as *españoles* (AGI, Lima, 301; Bowser 1974, 340).

The census results were a far cry from the reduction that the king, Phillip III, had demanded from colonial officials in 1608 when he ordered the viceroy "to stop the increase of these people [blacks, mulattoes, and mestizos]" so that "the land can be without the risks and dangers that they now pose and that can be expected from them in the future" (Konetzke 1958, 2:145). By 1636, a new *numeración* presented to Viceroy Marquis de Chinchón revealed that the colonial authorities had spectacularly failed to stem the increase of the black population. Lima then housed a total of 10,758 Spaniards, 13,620 blacks, and 861 mulattoes (AGI, Lima, 47; Bowser 1974, 341). Just as important, approximately one-quarter of those of African ancestry were classified as "free," a pattern that would increase with the passing of time. By the end of the eighteenth century, free Afro-Peruvians were slightly more numerous than slaves (Higgins 2005, 77; for the politics of slave manumission in Lima see Bowser 1974, 272–302; Jouve Martín 2009, 105–25). The only way to mitigate the perceived dangers was, as Viceroy

Marquis de Montesclaros had resignedly admitted in 1615, "to allow them to have their gatherings and dances in public spaces so that they can be watched, and to maintain as long as possible the separation of ethnic groups (*naciones*), for their diversity is what prevents them from joining in concerted action" (*Memorias de los virreyes*, 1859, 1: 31).[11]

The dual windfalls of Potosí's silver and the overseas slave trade accentuated the shortfalls of Lima's public health system. Slaves arrived in Lima after experiencing a strenuous journey under less than favourable physical conditions. Not surprisingly, many of them became sick and died shortly thereafter. City residents accused slaves of spreading all sorts of illnesses, the chief being leprosy, and the fear of contagion led to violence, with attacks against the enslaved as well as manumitted blacks (Warren 2004, 41–2). To alleviate the problem, the city council proposed in 1624 that a compound be built on the opposite side of the Rímac River to house newly arrived slaves so that the rest of the city's inhabitants could be spared the danger of contagion (Bowser 1974, 67). The new construction complemented the church and lazaretto that already existed in that area, which dated from 1563, when a certain Antón Sánchez had donated the land and the required funds (Barbagelata 1945, 57; Bravo de Lagunas y Castilla 1761, 46–7). Built under the invocation of San Lázaro, the hospital was an extremely modest, almost informal affair. Neither the initial funding nor the alms raised were sufficient to "bring the building to perfection or to accommodate more than two humble rooms close to the church as infirmaries" (ibid., 47).[12] Its main aim was to offer care for all those who suffered from leprosy, without distinguishing condition, sex, or age. It was not exclusively restricted to African slaves and free blacks, but it nevertheless became strongly associated with this section of the population (ibid., 73–4; Warren 2004, 40–4). Medical attention for sick slaves was supposed to be paid by their masters, but given that many slave owners either abandoned or manumitted their slaves to avoid covering the expenses associated with their care, the hospital administration assumed the costs, provided that if the slave recovered – which "only rarely happens," according to Lagunas y Castilla – he or she would become the property of the hospital (Bravo de Lagunas y Castilla 1761, 50).

By the mid-seventeenth century, the rising number of free blacks and mulattoes led to the construction of a separate hospital, the Hospital de San Bartolomé de los negros libres, which became a misnomer because

the hospital eventually also accepted slaves. Its origins date back to
1646, when the Jesuit priest Juan Perlín and the Augustinian friar Bartolomé de Vadillo decided to remedy the situation in which many elderly blacks found themselves. After a life of service to their masters,
they were "mercilessly thrown out of their homes and left to die of ex-
posure, since they were no longer useful for their owners" (Vargas
Machuca 1694, 11). Moved by compassion, Vadillo decided to build a
small structure in which freed slaves could receive physical and spiritual relief before they died.[13] Perlín and Vadillo's work was rewarded
in 1661, when Archbishop Pedro de Villagómez granted their request
to build a larger, more permanent hospital, which opened its doors on
25 March 1663, with the mission of providing blacks with protection,
medical assistance, and spiritual consolation. Despite the extraordinary
efforts of individuals like Perlín and Vadillo, most blacks and mulattoes
in Lima depended for their care not on the few doctors and surgeons
who worked in this and other city hospitals but on the many individuals who claimed to have access to a combination of natural and mag-
ical remedies.

Healers and Saints

Black slaves arriving in Lima brought with them African notions of
health and sickness that mixed with popular Spanish and Andean medical practices. The resulting body of knowledge was quickly adapted to
the urban environment by a wide variety of *curanderos* (healers),
hechiceros (sorcerers), and *ensalmadores* (those who cured by reciting
variations of biblical psalms) who populated the city of Lima. Both
newly arrived African folk healers and second- and third-generation
blacks and mulattoes frequently found themselves in competition with
their indigenous and Spanish counterparts, and soon earned a reputation for being able to treat all kinds of natural and supernatural illnesses (Garofalo 2006, 57–8). It was not only other slaves and poor city
dwellers who often turned to them in order to receive "specialized"
medical care. Even those who belonged to more affluent groups of society sought their help for solutions to health problems that educated
surgeons and doctors were frequently unable to solve (Cahill 1995,
125). This resulted in a paradox, observed by Lewis in her study on
witchcraft and caste in colonial Mexico: while many in the white elite

saw folk healers of African and indigenous descent as a source of remedies and medical care, colonial authorities considered them a danger to
public health, religious orthodoxy, and even the stability of the colony
(Lewis 2003). As Irene Silverblatt has put it, "heresy was a first step on
the slippery slope to treason" (2004, 150). Consequently, they were
persecuted, not by one but by two tribunals: the Tribunal del Protomedicato and the Tribunal de la Inquisición – the former condemning their practices as charlatanism and the latter characterizing their
actions as barbaric, superstitious, and idolatrous.

An example of such persecution was the case of Manuel de Jesús,
also known as Zaboga, a black man who was a slave in the Jesuit *hacienda* of San Juan. In 1733 he was condemned to appear in an *auto
de fe* by the Inquisition, where he was forced to carry a green candle in
his hands while wearing a dunce's cap and a rope around his neck. As
part of his punishment, Zaboga received two hundred lashes and was
banned from the city for six years. His crime had been to cast spells
using a combination of herbs, potions, and "indecent" body rubs, with
the purpose of advancing the illicit love affairs of his clients, along with
curing the physical pain caused by the curses he diagnosed. To this end,

> he used sacred words and objects, sacrilegiously invoked the
> saints' names for assistance and, making the sign of the cross with
> blessed palm branches, he ordered his patients to walk over them.
> He then rubbed their bodies with *cuyes* [guinea pigs] and gave
> them potions made of filthy water and powders that he feigned
> having acquired in the apothecary; he presented himself as some-
> one learned in medicine for having worked as a young man in
> the apothecary of the Jesuits, and through these lies he was able
> to obtain the amounts that he demanded. (Medina 1887, 2: 293)

Zaboga's case had been preceded by a large number of other trials
against *hechiceros* and *curanderos* of African descent. In 1570 a black
slave named Beatriz was brought to the Audiencia de Lima and accused
of being a "sorceress and invoker of demons" (Bowser 1974, 313).
That same year a mulatto was prosecuted for casting spells that prevented slave owners from mistreating blacks (AHN, Inquisición, 1027:
12r–12v). An Afro-Peruvian woman appeared in an *auto de fe* in 1592,
accused of invoking demons, the names of God and His Saints, and

preparing potions with sacramental bread, oil drops, blood, salt, and coriander (AHN, Inquisición, 1028: 231r–v; see also Iwasaki Cauti 1994, 160). In 1639 Luisa de Vargas, alias "Luisa la Cuarterona," was arrested by Inquisitorial authorities on charges of providing women with coca leafs that she had "moistened with *chicha* (corn whiskey)" so that they could obtain money and love from men (AHN, Inquisición, 1031: 349v). Remedies were not only for heartache but for other, more physical ailments as well. In the 1636 case against Bartolomé de Pradera, warden of the Inquisition's secret jail, the tribunal discovered that because of his lack of diligence, blacks had been able to bring into the cells "small balls, a little bit bigger than corn grains" that carried a strong odour of incense, and had instructed prisoners to take them as a sedative or painkiller "the night before they were to be tortured" (Medina 1887, 2:84). Determined in their pursuit, the Inquisition imposed harsh punishments on traditional healers (Newson 2006, 376). The most common sentence for most acts of "sorcery" was the whip. In a 1719 *auto de fe*, a black slave named Bernabé Morillo was forced to abjure *de vehementi* and was given 200 lashes for "having told women that they were cursed and offering to cure them, to take out the snakes and toads that were in their bodies, and to bring them good luck in their love affairs with men" (Medina 1887, 2:301). Physical punishment, however, was not the only way that colonial authorities kept healers and sorcerers in check. In 1719 a black woman named María Josefa Cangas, who had cast "such spells on her husband that made him lose his mind," was forced to abjure *de levi* and, possibly with the intention of putting her abilities towards a better end, condemned to "serve in a hospital for four years" (ibid.).

Yet not all black healers were persecuted, punished, or expelled from colonial Lima. Some of them successfully blended folk medicine and traditional beliefs with accepted medical and religious discourses. Perhaps no one exemplifies this better than Martín de Porres, a mulatto and a Dominican friar who was beatified in 1837 by Pope Gregory XVI and canonized by Pope John XXIII in 1962. Born in 1579 as the illegitimate son of a Spanish nobleman and a freed slave, Martín de Porres received a basic education. At the age of twelve, he began an apprenticeship with a barber-surgeon named Marcel de Rivero, who introduced him to the intricacies of his art. Soon afterwards, Martín de Porres entered the Dominican monastery of the Rosary as a *donado* (lay helper, or tertiary), becoming a coadjutor brother with an assignment to the monastery's infirmary. There he remained until his death, attending to the medical needs of the order's members as well as those of many other patients, who were attracted by his miraculous healing powers.

As with other traditional medical practitioners, Martín de Porres's healing methods combined commonly accepted seventeenth-century surgical techniques with religious and medical beliefs of African, Andean, and Peninsular origin. He was in charge of nearly every aspect of care, from administering purges and bloodletting to carrying out minor surgical operations. To this end, he employed some peculiar remedies to treat patients, utilizing hot bricks, egg whites, vinegar, syrups, and immersions in hot water. He washed his patients' wounds with wine and chewed rosemary, applied banana leaves, administered burned toad powder and water whipped with blood from a black rooster, and invoked the name of God and blessed his patients with the sign of the cross throughout treatment (Busto Durthurburu 2006, 118. See also Medina 1673; *Proceso de beatificación de San Martín de Porras* 1960).[14] In petitioning God and His Saints while administering treatment, Martín de Porres was walking a dangerous line. In 1629 the Inquisition had published an edict against "judiciary astrologers, chiromancers, sorcerers, and others of their kind" who made use of "vain and superstitious prayers, invoking our Lord God and the Holy Virgin, His Mother, and the Saints, and mixing in other improper invocations and words" (AHN Inquisición, 1040: 84v). Inquisition documents show that those who combined medicine and religion were frequently looked on with suspicion and investigated for propagating superstition, heresy, and sorcery. The colonial authorities routinely persecuted many *curanderos* who practised outside Lima, especially in the Andes, but also targeted licensed medical practitioners who claimed to have any sort of supernatural healing powers (Griffiths 1999, 185–97; Jouve Martín 2004, 181–98).

In spite of these persecutions, many of the witnesses who testified during the canonical investigation into the life and virtues of Martín de Porres stated that a crowd was always waiting for him at the door of his monastery to treat "abscesses and incurable wounds that medicinal drugs were unable to cure, and in just four days after Martín had laid his hands on them they improved and healed" (*Proceso* 1960, 124).

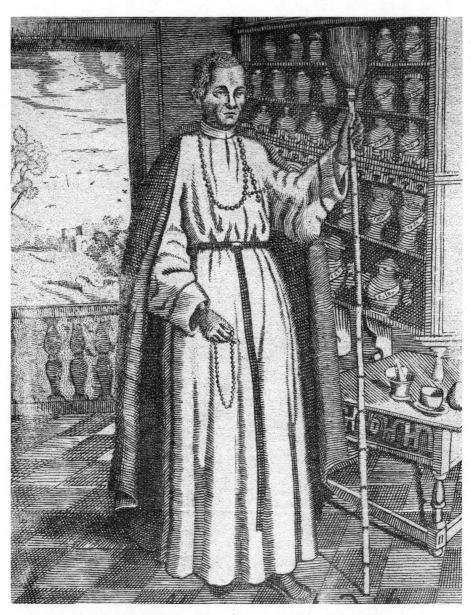

Saint Martin de Porres in his infirmary. A surgeon and a future saint, Martín de Porres blended religious and medical ideas from the European, indigenous, and African traditions in his medical practice.

Moreover, it was not only the destitute who sought Martin de Porres's help; even powerful figures were among his patrons. This was the case for Feliciano de la Vega, bishop of La Paz, who was closely linked to the campaigns aimed at the extirpation of idolatry and was therefore well versed in religious orthodoxy (Cussen 2005, 440–1). In 1639, finding himself in Lima on his way to Mexico, where he had been named archbishop, he suddenly fell ill. After the standard combination of bloodletting and other remedies proved ineffective, his doctors abandoned any hope of recovery. Moved by his suffering, his nephew urged him to call on Brother Martín and to ask him "to lay his hands" on wherever he felt pain. "I am confident," said his nephew, "that you will be immediately healed since I have been witness of the wonders that the Lord works through his hands in our monastery" (Medina 1673, 24). When Brother Martín finally appeared in front of the archbishop, "he laid his hand where the patient told him, and shortly afterwards the archbishop felt so free from the inopportune ailment and excessive pain that had afflicted him that one could say that Brother Martín had taken it away with his hand. The doctors who treated the archbishop were in awe and considered his recovery miraculous" (ibid., 25–6).

As the case of Martin de Porres also illustrates, blacks and especially mulattoes had already begun to make inroads in the lower echelons of the medical profession by the late sixteenth century. They were favoured by the chronic lack of properly trained physicians of Spanish origin and the fact that the members of the colonial elite preferred more profitable careers in law and the church to the prospect of becoming a surgeon or doctor. In a letter to the king in 1619, Viceroy Francisco de Borja y Aragón, Príncipe de Esquilache, expressed the colonial administration's general frustration with the continued shortage of trained medical practitioners and the resulting risks to public health: "This kingdom suffers in general from a great lack of doctors due to which barbers and Romance surgeons are now in charge of curing ailments, resulting in great harm to the population, and it is true that there are doctors who are allowed to practice and earn good money who do not know how to read or write" (quoted in Lastres 1951a, 88). In order to alleviate this situation and offer a much-needed service, the colonial authorities ignored the racial origins of those who practised surgery and medicine in Lima, provided they were the offspring of free and legitimate parents and could demonstrate adequate knowledge of their art. Lima's demographics ensured that they were for the most part of African descent, which in turn led to the growing and controversial presence of blacks and mulattoes in the Faculty of Medicine of the University of San Marcos.

Blacks and the Study of Medicine

Colonial medicine was an extraordinarily diverse and hierarchical profession. As Larrinaga pointed out in his *Apología de los cirujanos del Perú*, there were not only doctors and surgeons but also midwives, first nurses, second nurses, *barchilones*, *jeringueros*, and *untadores*, and so on. Even among surgeons, there was a clear hierarchy. The lower echelon was occupied by the *cirujanos flebotómicos* (phlebotomists), who were in charge of bloodletting and related services. They were followed by the *cirujanos romancistas* (Romance surgeons), whose limited knowledge of anatomy and medicine in general allowed them only to treat minor injuries. At the top were the *cirujanos latinos* (Latin surgeons). While little was needed in order to become a Romance surgeon or phlebotomist, becoming a Latin surgeon was an entirely different matter. These surgeons were authorized to perform emergency surgery and complicated procedures requiring skilful manipulation of the scalpel. They also had to demonstrate a knowledge of Latin – hence their name – in order to read medical and surgical treatises and interact with doctors and apothecaries on a daily basis (Romero 1942, 302). Even more crucially, Latin surgeons were required by the Protomedicato to attend classes at the University of San Marcos, train under the supervision of senior physicians, and pass a demanding exam before they could be granted their title and allowed to practise in the city hospitals.[15]

Despite being poorly remunerated, many free Afro-Peruvians considered the possibility of becoming a Romance or Latin surgeon an enticing prospect of upward social mobility. In fact, some of them aimed even higher. According to a report sent to Spain by Viceroy Marquís de Villagarcía, in 1737 a mulatto doctor presented himself as a candidate for the chair of Método de Galeno. Even though the viceroy swiftly rejected him on account of his race (*Memorias de los virreyes* 1859, 4: 480), his case illustrates the extent to which blacks and mulattoes had become a presence in Lima's medical world. Some of them were so visible as to be the object of satire in Juan del Valle y Caviedes's *Diente del*

Parnaso [*Tooth of Parnassus*] (1689), a collection of forty-seven poems ridiculing the physicians of Lima. Dedicated to "Death, Empress of Doctors," the book mentions by name some of the most famous physicians in the city. Valle y Caviedes directed some of his fiercest verses at Francisco Vargas Machuca, professor of Método de Galeno at the Universidad de San Marcos, whom he called "a cruel and inhuman hangman" of "barbarous ferocity," whose "remedies" had resulted in the death of Caviedes's cousin (Valle y Caviedes 1984, 60). Among the physicians who had African blood, Caviedes singled out the *zambo* surgeon Pedro de Utrilla, the son of a former slave of the same name, who had worked as a surgeon at the Hospital de Santa Ana (García Cáceres 1999, 90). In a *vejamen* (mock eulogy) dedicated to him "for having successfully removed a stone from a woman's body," Caviedes drew attention to Utrilla's racial origins and supposed lack of medical training by labelling him "Licentiate Black Pudding / and Bachelor Chimney," "Doctor of the Dark Room / of the Congo King of Guinea," and "runaway surgeon" (translation provided by Higgins 2005, 79).

Complaints about the presence of blacks and mulattoes in the medical profession did not take long to emerge. Already by 1701, some doctors and professors in the Faculty of Medicine at San Marcos found the increasing number of *castas* in their classes so frustrating that they asked the king "not to admit *mestizos, mulatos, zambos*, and *cuarterones* to any degree, since they were excluded as established in libro 1, titulo 22, art. 57 of the *Recopilación de leyes de las Indias*. They accused the university authorities of lack of zeal and of turning a blind eye on the racial origins and presumed illegitimacy of mulatto candidates. More crucially, they were able to gain the support of the viceroy and the royal prosecutor for their cause. To their suprise, the king's pronouncement came down against their request, noting that the aforementioned article of the *Recopilación* did not address the issue of race (see *Recopilación* 1841, 1: 138–9), and that Article 238 excluded from the university only "those with a note of infamy or who had been condemned by the Inquisition, as well as their sons and grandsons" (*Constituciones* 1735, 74). The expression "a note of infamy" was interpreted in this context as having to do with religion, illegitimate birth, or slavery, but not with race. Legitimate *mulatos* and *mestizos* born to free parents could therefore claim that the note of infamy did not refer to them, and consequently they were allowed to study surgery

or even medicine at San Marcos. As was frequently the case in the
Spanish empire, the king's word was rarely final, and the opposition to
the presence of blacks and *castas* at the Faculty of Medicine resurfaced
forty years later in the rarified social and political context that followed
the devastating earthquake of 1746.

By then, the massive influx of African slaves that had been charac-
teristic of the seventeenth century had somewhat subsided, but the city
of Lima had not turned "whiter." The colonial census of 1700 had
seemed to give some respite to those who were generally worried about
the growth of the *castas*. It showed – albeit somewhat misleadingly –
that the Afro-Peruvian population of the city had been reduced to
approximately one-third of the city's total population, compared with
1636, when Afro-Peruvians had accounted for over one-half of the
city's inhabitants. The census listed 4,063 individuals classified as *indios*, 3,370 as *mulatos*, and 7,659 as *negros*, against 19,632 classified
as *españoles* (*Numeración general* 1985 [1700]; Pérez Cantó, 1982,
390). A closer look reveals, however, a somewhat different picture.
Since the key racial category of *mestizos* was not counted in the census,
it seems legitimate to conclude that the number of those classified as *españoles* must have included many *mestizos* and was therefore exag-
gerated. Also, the census, which aimed to give the colonial authorities
an idea of the number of "able" hands in the city in case it needed to
be defended against foreign attack, did not provide a racial breakdown
of those living in monasteries, convents, and hospitals. Since these institutions were the major holders of slaves and servants in the Peruvian
capital, it is likely that the proportion of blacks and mulattoes was significantly understated.

The census compiled by Viceroy Francisco Gil de Taboada y Lemos
in 1790 offered a much more complete picture. Purportedly "the most
accurate and truthful numeration" ever made in Lima, it estimated the
total population of the city to be 52,627 ("Reflexiones históricas y
políticas" 1791, 93).[16] According to its calculations, the capital of the
viceroyalty of Peru had a total of 17,215 *españoles*, 3,912 *indios*, 4,631
mestizos, 8,960 *negros*, 5,972 *mulatos*, 2,383 *cuarterones*, 219 *quinterones*, 3,384 *zambos*, and 1,120 *chinos* (AGI, Indiferente, 1527
[Lima, 5 December 1790]). When taken together, Afro-Peruvian *castas*
– that is, *negros, mulatos, cuarterones, quinterones*, and *zambos* – still
constituted the majority of the population. And when other *castas* were

added to the mix, such as *indios, mestizos,* and *chinos,* those who claimed to be of a purely Spanish lineage found themselves again in a minority. The situation must have been similar on the night of 28 October 1746, when a devastating earthquake struck Lima and the port of Callao.

The tremors destroyed most of the city's buildings and seriously affected its sanitary infrastructure. The damage to hospitals and other health installations was enormous, and its impact lasted at least until the close of the colonial period (Cahill 1995, 151–2). Almost coincidentally, "a marked apprehension of the black in the Universities and in the professions appeared in the Spanish Empire, especially in Lima and the Caribbean" (Lanning 1985, 183). These were not just academic and professional anxieties; there was the fear that blacks and the indigenous population might rebel against the colonial order as they had done in the Lima Conspiracy and Huarochirí Rebellion (Walker 2008, 156–85). Against the background of a devastated city and faced with the growing threat of the *castas* to the status quo, the colonial authorities finally decided to restore order and in 1750 granted the white physicians of Lima what they had been requesting since 1701.

That year, Viceroy Conde de Superunda prohibited "the admission of *mestizos, zambos,* mulattoes, and quadroons to the University in Lima" (King 1951, 433; *Memorias de los virreyes* 1859, 480). On 27 September 1752, King Ferdinand VI sided with his viceroy and issued a royal decree "to put an end to all controversies and establish a rule for the future," in which he made clear, once and for all, that those with "any note of infamy" such as *mestizos, zambos, mulatos* and *cuarterones,* were not allowed to study at the university. The prohibitions went even further when the king declared null and void any university degrees obtained by individuals of those castes who "had been admitted to and graduated from the university, especially in the Faculty of Medicine, owing to the lack of diligence of those who had governed it" (ibid.). In the eyes of the higher colonial administration, the decadence of the university and of medicine itself had been in no small part a consequence of the failure to require certificates of blood purity from students upon matriculation (Lanning 1985, 184; Warren 2010, 61). The royal decree took this issue seriously and established a standard administrative practice wherein "prospective students at San Marcos be asked whether they belong to any of the four castes, as is commonly done in the process of becoming a notary, during which candidates are asked whether they are mulattoes" (*Memorias de los virreyes* 1859, 4:480–1).

The measures adopted by the Count of Superunda and King Ferdinand VI found a receptive audience among many white doctors and high colonial bureaucrats. They were echoed by Viceroy Manuel Amant y Yunient, who replaced the Count of Superunda in 1761. In his *Memoria de Gobierno*, he expressed his determination to redeem the practice of medicine and the University of San Marcos "from despicable and vile characters, stopping *infames* or individuals of bad reputation from graduating, particularly in medicine, which is the one subject they have favoured the most in reducing this noble faculty to its present decay" (*Memorias de los virreyes* 1859, 4:479).

Many Afro-Peruvians who aspired to pursue a career in medicine may have felt dismayed at the almost insurmountable obstacles raised by the royal decree and the viceregal administration, but they were not dissuaded from trying and they found ways to circumvent the existing legislation. They also found an unexpected source of support in Hipólito Unanue and those who considered the development of surgery and the renovation of the medical sciences as key for the future of the viceroyalty. Such was the case with José Manuel Valdés and José Manuel Dávalos who, together with Larrinaga, became the most famous black physicians of the late colonial period.

Mulatto Physicians and *Criollo* Reformers

On 29 July 1767, in a poor house near the convent of Santa Clara, José Manuel Valdés was born to Baltasar Valdés, a mestizo musician from Saña, and María Cabada, a mulatto woman.[17] Valdés was especially fortunate because his mother's employers, a relatively well-positioned Spanish couple that owned an apothecary in the centre of the city, became his godparents (Lavalle n.d., 2). When he was three, his mother placed him in the *miga*, as it was customary to call elementary school. Soon afterwards, the teacher informed Valdés's parents that she could not teach her young pupil anything more, since the boy had already learned the entire school curriculum; apparently, he was able to read and write at a basic level and knew the fundamentals of Christian doctrine by heart (ibid., 2–3). For many young mulattoes, this was the point at which their education ended and they were considered ready to learn a trade and enter into a contract of apprenticeship. Fortunately for Valdés, his godparents realized that he was intellectually gifted and offered to give him "a more elevated and complete education than the one that corresponded to his caste" (ibid., 3). Valdés was then admitted to the Augustinian school of San Ildenfonso, where he studied "all the sciences and subjects of his curriculum with distinction, excelling so much in theology and Latin that he became proficient in writing and speaking in the language of Horatius" (ibid.). According to his biographers, Valdes' aspiration was to become a doctor, but the limitations imposed by the Royal Decree of 1752 convinced him that the only way to practise medicine was to become a surgeon. He began his career at the Hospital de San Andrés, one of five major hospitals that existed in late-eighteenth-century Lima, under the supervision of Juan de la Roca, a reputed Spanish doctor, who recommended him to Hipólito Unanue.

In 1788, at the age of twenty-one and after having completed a five-year internship at San Andrés, Valdés received the degree of Latin Surgeon and the authorization to practise surgery from the Royal Protomedicato, then chaired by Dr Juan José de Aguirre (Lastres 1951b, 131). Valdés's proficiency with a scalpel did not go unnoticed by the general public,[18] and Unanue, already a renowned physician, frequently requested that the mulatto surgeon replace him whenever a patient was in grave danger, saying with a mixture of admiration and condescension: "Tell José Manuel to come here to do his witchcraft" (Lavalle, 5). Owing to his fame as a surgeon and thanks to the testimonials provided by Juan de la Roca and Hipólito Unanue, Valdés received temporary permission from the Protomedicato to practise medicine. Technically, the Protomedicato's authorization was for one year only, but "Valdés practices so skillfully that no one remembers that his license has expired, and for fifteen years he practices as a full fledged doctor" (Romero 1942, 302).

Finally, on 11 June 1806, King Charles IV signed a *real cédula* freeing José Manuel Valdés from the limitations imposed by the Royal Decree of 1752. Valdés obtained his bachelor's degree with a thesis in which he passionately defended the value of surgery in the practice of medicine. Publishing it under the title *Theses medicae pro gradus licenciatus obteniendo*, he dedicated the essay to Viceroy José Fernando

Abascal y Sousa, who had arrived in Lima the year before (Valdés 1807, 1). Valdés was allowed to take the doctoral exams just a few days after having defended his *Theses medicae* in view of his vast experience in the treatment of patients and on account of the written support of doctors Hipólito Unanue and Juan de la Roca. According to Lavalle, he answered the questions posed by his doctoral tribunal "with such energy that he demonstrated and made known his aptitude, suitability, resourcefulness, and recognized talent, for which he was approved by acclamation and without need for a vote" (Lavalle n.d., 8). The practical part of the exam took place under the supervision of Dr Miguel Tafur who, after witnessing Valdés complete the required medical rounds at the Hospital del Espíritu Santo, informed the *Protomedicato* that he had demonstrated "the sound judgment and reflection that characterize an accomplished practitioner" (ibid., 8–9).

Not all mulattoes, however, were willing to wait twenty years before they were recognized as doctors. As it was, the text of the Royal Decree of 1752 prohibited individuals of African ancestry from attending the Faculty of Medicine at San Marcos or at any other university in Spain or Spanish America. But it did not discuss or even acknowledge the possibility of mulattoes becoming doctors elsewhere. The Peninsular authorities may have thought it too unlikely that anyone with African blood would ever leave Lima to study medicine, but that was exactly what José Manuel Dávalos did. The legitimate child of Joaquín Dávalos, a Spanish nobleman of some means, and María Samudio, a black woman, Dávalos was born in Lima in 1758. He first studied at the Seminario conciliar de Santo Toribio, and then – like Valdés – at the Augustinian school of San Ildefonso (Lastres 1951a, 265–6).[19] After graduating as *bachiller* in 1780, Dávalos decided to study surgery and anatomy under Dr Francisco de Rúa y Collazos at the Hospital de San Andrés. In 1784, wanting to become a doctor but unable to fulfill his desire in Lima because of the restrictions posed by the royal decree, Dávalos resolved to use his relatively modest family fortune to continue his education in France at the University of Montpellier, which had a medical faculty of international renown. Once there, he became acquainted with the works of Lavoisier in chemistry, Chaptal in clinical medicine, and Fourcroy in therapeutics, among others, and was able to complete his doctorate with the thesis *De morbis nonnullis Limae grassantibus ipsorumque therepeia* [On some common illnesses in Lima and their therapy], which was published in Montpellier in 1787.

Shortly after its publication, Dávalos returned to Peru, where the Viceroy Teodoro de Croix assigned him a position as a professor in chemistry at San Marcos with a salary of 1,200 pesos. The position lasted just one year, during which Dávalos was unable to start teaching "as His Excellency had mandated, because there are a thousand difficult obstacles to overcome" (Dávalos 1810, 9). According to Lastres, some accused the mulatto doctor of plagiarizing previous works, and they were opposed to recognizing his French title unless he paid the full fees for becoming a doctor in Lima (Lastres 1955, 158–9). In 1795 Dávalos applied for the chair in Botany, offering to teach the subject free of charge "while they obtain funding for the chair" (Dávalos 1810, 11), an almost irresistible offer to the public treasury (Goicoetxea Marcaida 1989, 645). He was awarded the position and began making arrangements to teach the subject by preparing the course program, writing an inaugural discourse, and even hiring a gardener "for the Royal Garden at San Andrés that the administration had provisionally assigned to me, who sows and cultivates the plants that I request with great effort and expense" (Dávalos 1810, 12). Unfortunately, his academic opponent, Juan Tafalla, presented a complaint, and Dávalos was dispossessed of the chair.[20] In sheer desperation, Dávalos considered leaving Lima for good: "Wanting to establish my home where fate would be less adverse, I have decided to move to the Mexican viceroyalty" (ibid., 13). In 1798, however, Dávalos tried his luck once more by presenting his candidacy to the chair of Método de Medicina, which had been left vacant after Cosme Bueno's death. Instead, the chair went to Miguel Tafur, a rising star in Lima's medical world who would become protomédico after independence. Dávalos eventually became substitute chair of Vísperas de Medicina in 1806, and it was only after the foundation of the Real colegio de medicina y cirugía de San Fernando in 1810 that he finally obtained a stable faculty position as professor of Materia médica.

In addition to Valdés, Dávalos, and Larrinaga, there were other Afro-Peruvians who became well-known physicians in late colonial Lima even though they did not leave a comparable record. Of these, Manuel Atanasio Fuentes considered Faustos, Montero, Puente, and Dávila to be among the most distinguished (Fuentes 1985 [1866], 170).

José Santos Montero was active as a surgeon in the hospitals of San Bartolomé and San Andrés as well as in the *pardo* civic calvary unit (Pamo Reina 63, 2009). According to Atanasio Fuentes, "nature seemed to have destined him for that profession [surgery]; for instead of the huge and horny hands that are generally a mark of men of the negro race, his were small, delicate, and soft as those of a *señorita*. His sight was keen and his hand steady even at the age of sixty. He acquired by means of his constant efforts and long studies such skill in the most delicate and difficult operations that foreign surgeons who have known him were astonished to see him so well acquainted with the progress of surgery and so expert in the use of the most recently invented instruments" (Fuentes 1985 [1867], 167. See also Nemesio Vargas 1910, 85).

José María Dávila was described in 1812 as being a "professor of medicine and surgery in this city" and one of the first to lecture in the Royal Amphitheatre about *carbunclo* (anthrax). Apparently, he tried, but failed, to become chair of Clínica at San Marcos, a setback attributed not to his shortcomings but to the fact that the public did not hold "his talents in the high regard that they deserved" (*Colección de los discursos* 1812, 106n26). As for José Puente, he was portrayed that same year as being an excellent diagnostician with a rare gift "for perceiving the hidden causes of illnesses" and having an unsurpassed capacity for understanding their development and the remedies needed to combat them (ibid.). Regarding Mariano Faustos, Larrinaga described him as an able Romance surgeon, well versed in Latin and philosophy, who was active in the Hospital de San Bartolomé from 1789 until his death in 1801 (Larrinaga 1791, 33). And, Valdizán singled out the black surgeons Jerónimo and Miguel Utrilla, descendants of those mentioned by Caviedes in his *Diente del Parnaso*. According to Valdizán, Jerónimo de Utrilla became widely admired for having "an exceptional gift for prognosis" that allowed him to become "master even among masters," in spite of not being able to explain his conclusions properly, "due to a lack of eloquency" (Valdizán 1929, 3: 5–6).

All these physicians were active at a time when the teaching and practice of medicine was experiencing a profound transformation in the viceroyalty of Peru.[21] The changes started in the mid-eighteenth century under the leadership of the doctor, mathematician, and cosmographer Cosme Bueno. A native of Spain, Bueno had arrived in Peru in 1730. He became chair of Método de Galeno at San Marcos shortly after obtaining his doctorate in medicine in 1750. This did not prevent him from being appointed First Cosmographer of the Realm and chair of Mathematics at the University of San Marcos in 1758 (Moreno 1872, 7). From that privileged academic position, Bueno lectured on Cartesian philosophy, Newtonian phyisics, and the ideas of Thomas Sydenham and Herman Boerhaave in medicine. At a time when, as his biographer Gabriel Moreno put it, the study of medicine in Peru "was reduced to being purely Peripatetic" (1872, 6), Bueno sought to modernize the curriculum, especially the teaching of anatomy. He introduced Martín Martínez's *Anatomía completa del hombre* (1728) as the main anatomical textbook in his classes, a provocative work that severely criticized those physicians who "after forty years of practice leave this life without having ever seen an anatomical dissection" (Martínez 1752 [1728], xxiv).[22] Larrinaga himself studied surgery under Bueno's supervision and fondly recalled his teaching and the importance he attributed to the practical study of anatomy over purely theoretical approaches:

> Doctor Cosme Bueno, who is not inferior in science, erudition, and glory to all the Newtons and Boerhaaves of the world, did not want me to study any work other than Martínez's *Anatomía completa*, not only because it is very appropriate for its philosophical character, but also because it deals with the issues that are most essential and necessary for knowledge of the sick, healthy, or dead body. This wise doctor, who was fond of me and was so kind as to teach me my first theoretical lessons in this faculty, chose Martínez's book over Heister's, Juan de Dios López's, and the great Winslow's, who was known among the French as the Prince of Modern Anatomy. (Larrinaga 1791, 14–15)

Bueno's reformist zeal survived in the rising figure of Hipólito Unanue. Born in Arequipa in 1753, Unanue moved to Lima in 1777. By 1789, he had already obtained the chair of Anatomy at San Marcos and immediately began to press for the modernization of the teaching of medicine in Peru and the creation of an anatomical amphiteatre.[23] This project became a reality three years later, on 21 December 1792. In his inaugural speech, "Decadencia y restauración del Perú" [Decadence and restoration of Peru], Unanue set out to explain his medical and social agenda. He linked the economic and political decadence of the viceroyalty to the destitute condition that characterized the teaching and practice of medicine. This decadence was in turn a major reason for the "depopulation" of Peru and the loss of its economic potential. The disregard that colonial authorities had shown for medicine and particularly for anatomy was what had "ruined our towns, desolated our fields, and destroyed our mines, consuming the generous hands that promoted their splendour, fecundity, and riches" (Unanue 1792, 92). Unanue envisioned that the teaching of anatomy, the reform of surgery, and the progress of medicine would bring his *patria*, Peru, to a "blissful age" when "with the multiplication of the population, its old villages, towns, and cities would remain standing and would be extended and improved; the canals built by the Incas would be preserved and new ones opened so that water from the Andes could increase the flow of rivers, and these in turn could be used to irrigate its vast fields" (ibid., 125).

Unfortunately, the presence of an earlier generation of scholars formed by doctors such as Juan de Aguirre (chair of Prima de Medicina and protomédico from 1784), Francisco Ruia (chair of Visperas de Medicina from 1785), and Marcelino Alzamora (chair of Método de Medicina from 1787) "effectively stopped him by holding until 1807 the very chairs controlling the possibility of reform. Until these men moved, the founding of a renovated medical school was utterly impossible, for each one chose not to cooperate with Unanue" (Woodham 1970, 704). In preparation for that time and in order to break their resistance, Unanue forged alliances with those who shared similar views of medicine and country. Unlike many of his predecessors, he saw surgery as a fundamental part of medicine and not as a secondary art. Consequently, he sought to enlist the help of surgeons who, like Valdés and Larrinaga, were on the front lines of medical care in Lima and embodied in his eyes the tranformation that the discipline had experienced since the mid-eighteenth century.

The fact that Unanue included individuals of African origin in his projects speaks to his open and scientifically minded attitude on social and scientific issues, but it should not lead us to believe that he and other reform-minded physicians saw black surgeons and doctors as their equals. White doctors did not hesitate to affirm their perceived social and racial superiority and, as Dávalos had learned, their preeminence in the competition for academic positions. Despite this, there can be no doubt that white physicians actively supported and promoted the work of their black peers whom they considered particularly gifted. In this regard, Unanue used the clinical lecture series that he had established at the anatomical amphitheatre "as a platform to help mulatto colleagues advance their careers (of the first seven lecturers, four – Dávalos, Valdés, J.M. Dávila and José Puente – were mulattoes)" (Glick 1991, 323). As we shall see in the next chapter, he went even further. He paved the way for two men of African ancestry – Valdés and Larrinaga – to publish their medical findings in what soon became the most important political and scientific publication of the colonial Enlightenment: the *Mercurio peruano*.

CHAPTER 2

Enlightened Surgeons, Public Writers

Unanue considered Valdés's and Larrianaga's expertise as an example of the radical improvement that surgery had experienced in eighteenth-century Lima compared with earlier times, when it was known "only by name" in Peru (Unanue 1793a, 106–7; Haenke 1901, 83).[1] Progress in the field had been linked to French anatomical and surgical advances in the late seventeenth century. French surgery became notably more influential in the Spanish empire after the arrival of the Bourbon dynasty on the Spanish throne in 1701.[2] Also following the French example, the Spanish Crown created surgical colleges in Cádiz, Madrid, and Barcelona that served as models in the colonies. In New Spain chairs of anatomy and surgery were established in Mexico City in 1767, and during the next decade Mexican surgeons successfully lobbied colonial and metropolitan authorities to establish a school of surgery completely independent of the university and the Protomedicato (Burke 1977, 64). In Peru, however, change came at a considerably slower pace. Established in 1711, the chair in Anatomy at San Marcos did not become functional until the mid-eighteenth century. The construction of an anatomical amphitheatre was postponed until the 1790s, and an independent school of medicine and surgery did not exist until the 1810s.

Despite the general lack of resources, the influence of French surgeons in the viceroyalty of Peru was felt early on, as illustrated by the case of Pablo Petit. He arrived in Lima in 1723 after having been approved to practise medicine by the two royal courts of Paris and Madrid and designated "Surgeon in Chief [cirujano mayor] of the artillery and hospitals of the armies of His Catholic Majesty in Catalonia" (Petit 1723, title page). While serving in Spain, Petit had published a brief treatise on childbirth entitled *Cuestiones generales sobre el modo de partear y cuidar a las mujeres que están embarazadas o paridas* (1717). Shortly after arriving in Peru, he published an essay devoted to cancer, *Epístola oficiosa sobre esencia y curación del cáncer, vulgarmente llamado Zaratán* (1723), and seven years later he penned a treatise on syphilis, *Breve tratado de la enfermedad venerea o mal gálico* (1730). Petit's ambition – which was later reflected in Valdés's and Larrianga's works – was to elevate surgery in Peru from the category of a despised art to that of a rigorous science. To this end, he did not hesitate to compare surgery to mathematics:

> I call surgery an Art just to stay true to its etymology since the word is composed of two Greek terms: "Keir," which means "hand," and "Ergot," which means "operation." Therefore, a surgeon is someone who "operates" with his "hands" … but since the hand does not do anything other than what reason dictates, surgery deserves the title of science no less than mathematics, since mathematicians also need [to use their hands] to draw on paper the figures and demonstrations devised by their understanding. (Petit 1723, n.p.)

Not everyone in Lima shared the scientific ambitions of Petit and agreed with the new status accorded to surgery in the Spanish empire. A particularly good example of the animosity towards surgeons was the *Causa médico-criminal* taken up in 1764 by the protomédico Hipólito Bueno de la Rosa and some professors of medicine at San Marcos against the surgeons, apothecaries, and phlebotomists in the city of Lima. Proponents of the *Causa* sought to ensure that such practitioners would be "contained in the terms of their professions" and denounced the flagrant abuses perpetrated by surgeons who, "having overextended their practice beyond what their instruction allows and the faculties that Your Excellency has conceded to them, have practised medicine with total impunity and have caused known damage in treating dangerous internal illnesses and taking care of extremely difficult medical cases with such grave and ill-fated consequences that it is not licit to explain them" (Bueno de la Rosa 1764, 1r). Responsibility for these actions, they maintained, rested not only upon overconfident surgeons but also upon "some doctors who, renouncing their honour and despising the prerogatives of their profession, in light of the corruption that has occurred, defend them and encourage them to the odious point that they consult each other" (ibid.). Bueno de la Rosa's words were echoed by others, such as Isidro Joseph Ortega y Pimentel, chair of Método de Galeno at San Marcos, who in his *Oración conminatoria* – a discourse published together with the *Causa médico-criminal* – lamented that "the imaginary successes with which some of these surgeons have achieved a position of honour have been darkened by the myriad corpses with which their impiety has filled the horrors of the sepulchre" (ibid., 20r).

The actions of both Bueno de la Rosa and Ortega y Pimentel were motiviated by a desire to protect their professional status. As surgery began to realize its potential for alleviating physical illnesses, its practitioners often overstepped the profession's boundaries and worked in areas traditionally reserved for medicine (Burke 1977, 34). It is also likely that they saw their *Causa médico-criminal* and *Oración conminatoria* as a way of keeping individuals of African descent – who, as Larrinaga pointed out in his *Apología*, constituted an important part of the city's surgeons – from meddling in a profession that the Royal Decree of 1752 had declared exclusively white. Unanue himself was not oblivious to these preoccupations and fought to keep surgeons firmly under the control of doctors. But unlike the contempt that Bueno de la Rosa and Ortega y Pimentel showed for their less fortunate colleagues, Unanue saw the advancement of surgery and the study of anatomy as a fundamental part of his efforts at medical reform. Consequently, he gave José Pastor de Larrinaga and José Manuel Valdés – who by then had become two of the most prominent surgeons in Lima – the possibility of expressing their ideas in the pages of the *Mercurio peruano*, one of the most important journals of the Spanish American Enlightenment.[3]

The role of the *Mercurio peruano* as a vehicle for the promotion of science and social reform has long been acknowledged by historians (Clément 1997; Meléndez 2006, 207–27). The fact that Unanue used the journal to promote the works of individuals of African ancestry such as Larrinaga and Valdés has, however, eluded many of them. This can be explained by a combination of two facts: on the one hand, the journal's policy on the use of pseudonyms in order to conceal the author's identity; and, on the other, the scientific nature of their contributions. In this regard, their texts were virtually indistinguishable from those of their white peers and did not constitute an attempt to articulate a discourse on race or develop a form of self-conscious "black writing." They were chosen by Unanue not because of their *casta* but because they embodied in his eyes the progress experienced by surgery in the eighteenth century and because they shared his reformist agenda. For their part, both surgeons adopted as their own the objectives that had led to the founding of the journal: the promotion of science and reform throughout the viceroyalty of Peru and the Spanish empire as a whole. In line with this aim, they tried to make their knowledge accessible to non-specialists even when commenting on elaborate surgical techniques. But it was not only surgery in which they were interested. Both used the *Mercurio peruano* to express their opinon on various social and philosophical issues. Larrinaga even sought to develop his literary persona by submitting historical poems on the royal lineage of the Incas and the establishment of colonial rule in Peru. They saw the opportunity to publish in the *Mercurio peruano* as a fundamental part of a process of self-fashioning that allowed them to transcend their role as physicians in order to become public intellectuals in Lima's world of letters.

Writing for the *Mercurio peruano*

The *Mercurio peruano de historia, literatura y noticias públicas* was published in Lima between 1791 and 1795. Its founding members, in addition to Hipólito Unanue, included such prominent Peruvian intellectuals as José Rossi y Rubí, José L. Egaña, and Demetrio Guasque. In 1787 they had formed a group known as the Academia filarmónica, or the Philharmonic Academy (Clément 1997, 22; Dager Alva 2001, 98). The academy's main aim was to discuss science, literature, and politics in an atmosphere of friendship and learning, working towards the common goal of Peru's advancement. The atmosphere of optimism and friendship that dominated those first meetings was captured in an article that later appeared in one of *Mercurio peruano*'s first issues: "Oh,

Lima! If you knew of the sweetness that the union of a literary gathering brings with it you would be far from division and tumult ... Motherland of so many learned individuals, your population would be happy if you added some of your many enlightened citizens to the gathering of the Philharmonic Youth" ("Historia de la sociedad académica" 1791, 50). Unfortunately, unforeseen personal circumstances led to the temporary dissolution of the group: "*Homótimo* [Demetrio Guasque] went to the court, where he was called to a career in politics; *Hesperófilo* [José Rossi y Rubi], having lost the most precious and wonderful thing he had in the world, left for the mountains to mitigate the pain of the loss; *Hermágoras* [José L. Egaña] was pained by the loss of these two companions; *Aristio* [Unanue] fell sick; *Mindírido* got married; and that's how the Philarmonic Academy disappeared in an instant, in everything but name" (ibid.).

After a hiatus of a little more than a year and a half, the group came together again under the name Sociedad académica de Amantes del País. Modelled on the metropolitan Sociedades de Amantes del País, the Sociedad académica was established as an academic and philanthropic institution, based on Enlightenment principles and devoted to the advancement of the arts and sciences as well as to the cause of social reform in Peru. As its secretary, Unanue took a leading role in the new society and urged its members to put their ideas in writing. The publication of Jaime Bausate's ill-fated *Diario curioso* convinced the members that in Lima's public sphere there was "a substantial void for the subjects generated by our academic discussions" (ibid.). In their efforts to fill this void, they enlisted the help of Jacinto Calero y Moreira, a lawyer in the Real Audiencia, who became the main editor of the *Mercurio peruano*, and without whom "the works of the *Sociedad de Amantes del País* might have remained buried in the forgotten past, as happened with the Philharmonic" (ibid.). As a result of the combined efforts of this group of intellectuals, the first issue of the *Mercurio peruano* appeared on 2 January 1791. Most of the articles published in the journal – around 33%, according to Jean-Pierre Clement – were related to history and geography. Scientific articles ranked second, accounting for approximately 25% of the total number of contributions. The importance of medicine in the *Mercurio* is reflected by the fact that, of the scientific articles, the vast majority dealt with medical issues (64%), followed by natural history (21%), physics (10%), and chem-

istry (10%) (Clement 1997, 95–8). University professors, high-ranking colonial bureaucrats, and learned members of the church were
among those who contributed to the journal most frequently. On the
topic of medicine, seven authors accounted for nearly all of the journal's articles on the subject. Leaving aside those written by Unanue,
who was the most prolific author in the *Mercurio peruano*, many of the
medical articles were written by José Manuel Valdés and José Pastor
Larrinaga.[4]

The two mulatto surgeons were also the only individuals of African
ancestry who wrote for the *Mercurio*, which was dominated by members of the white colonial elite. Their inclusion should not lead us to believe that the *Mercurio peruano* was directed by a radical group of
intellectuals who railed against racial prejudice and championed the
cause of social equality. The editors certainly wanted to improve conditions for black slaves and freemen, but they were focused on gradual
reform, not necessarily on revolutionary change and even less on abolition. Nonetheless, Joseph Rossi y Rubí did not hesitate to call blacks
"brothers" and to denounce the situation that many African slaves
faced in Peru's *haciendas*: "These unhappy sons of the Almighty, our
own brothers through the incontrovertible lineage of Adam ... are
found reduced to the level of a bundle of goods and are sometimes
treated worse than the donkeys found in the same estates that they irrigate with their sweat" (Rossi y Rubi 1791, 113). Despite these compassionate words, the general opinion held by most contributors to the
Mercurio concerning Afro-Peruvians was ambivalent at best, with
many considering them "an emblem of disorder and a dubious group
due to their lack of education" (Meléndez 2006, 213). Joseph Ignacio
de Lequanda, a high-ranking officer of the Real hacienda and an occa-
sional contributor to the journal, expressed what could be considered
the prevailing view about blacks and mulattoes. In his articles,
Lequanda wrote of his general contempt for free blacks as "a union of
disobedient individuals" who were "common perpetrators of murders,
robberies, and the most criminal excesses" (Lequanda 1793, 49). He regarded mulattoes as the "gypsies of the Americas" because of their sim-
ilarity in skin colour as well as their wit and resourcefulness, and
warned readers that "just as the fields produce good and bad weeds, in
this lineage we also find many bad individuals and a few good ones"
(Lequanda 1794, 115). Among the few good mulattoes, he conceded,

were "bright people loyal to the king and to the Spaniards" who had
been able to excel in various professions, such as "tailors, cobblers,
barbers, button-makers, tobacconists, agriculturalists, silversmiths, car-
penters, architects, blacksmiths, ribbon-makers, and many other valuable professions throughout the city" (ibid.). As trained and successful
surgeons, Larrinaga and Valdés were no doubt seen in this slightly more
favourable light by many of those involved in the publication of the
Mercurio peruano.

The publication of their texts was also facilitated by the journal's
editorial policy on authorship. Calero y Moreira had already warned
readers that it was not important "to know the name and circumstances of those who work on the *Mercurio* with me. By their works
these men can be characterized; and these are always substantial, when
they are not delinquent" (Calero y Moreira 1790, 7). Contributors
wcrc therefore asked – although not necessarily obligated – to use pseudonyms instead of their real names. Accordingly, Unanue signed his
pieces as Aristio, José Rossi y Rubí as Hesperiófilo, José L. Egaña as
Hermágoras, and Demetrio Guasque as Homotimo. The two mulatto
surgeons also employed this strategy in order to disguise their identites.
José Manuel Valdés adopted the *nom de plume* Erisistrato Svadel; "Erisistrato" was an obvious reference to the Greek physician and
anatomist Erasistratus (304–250 BCE), and "Svadel," was an anagram
of his last name, "Valdés." Larrinaga chose to sign as José Torpás de
Ganarrila, a pseudonym formed from his first name ("José") and the
syllables of his two last names written in reverse order: "Torpás" (Pastor) and "Ganarrila" (Larrinaga). The fact that their pen names barely
concealed their real ones illustrates that the use of pseudonyms was
more a literary game than evidence of any serious attempt to hide their
identities. While it may have helped to keep their identities a mystery
for overseas subscribes, everyone in Lima's extremely small intellectual
world must have known who Svadel and José Torpás de Ganarrila were
and to what *casta* they belonged. Nevertheless, their real names and
racial labels were deliberately omitted in publication so that science
could take its proper place and free discussion could flourish. They
were invited to contribute to the *Mercurio peruano* because their work
as Latin surgeons had placed them on the front lines of medical care in
colonial Lima and not as representatives of a particular racial group.
There was, nevertheless, a limit to how open the editors were willing

to be on the issue of race, and despite their contributions to the journal, neither Valdés nor Larrinaga were invited to become members of the exclusive, all-white group of intellectuals who formed the Sociedad académica de Amantes del país.[5]

The Science and Practice of Surgery

Most of the texts Valdés and Larrinaga submitted to the *Mercurio peruano* dealt with the anatomical and practical observations they had made during their practice. Valdés expressed his position on the state of the surgical sciences in Lima at the end of the eighteenth century in his article "Sobre las utilidades de la anatomía comprobadas con una observación" [On the usefulness of anatomy, proved with an observation] (Valdés 1792b), in which he illustrated the relevance of postmortem anatomical examinations for the advancement of medicine in general and surgery in particular. Following the teachings of Viennese physician Anton de Haen, he considered autopsies not only as a way of illustrating "the admirable organization of living bodies" but also a fundamental tool for revealing "the hidden causes of a man's death, which even the shrewdest observer is not always able to predict" (Valdés 1792b, 183).

In order to illustrate this, Valdés described the case of a certain Pedro Bustamante, a black slave from the Cambunda region in Angola. At about forty years of age, Pedro had died after being accidentally hit while taking part in a dance called *Lumbé* with other members of his *nación*, or ethnic group (ibid., 184). Emphasizing the distance that separated him – an educated surgeon – from Lima's black slaves in spite of their shared African heritage, Valdés described *Lumbé* as a dance "suitable for blacks [*propio de negros*]," having "the same irregularities as all dances of such people, it being very common for participants to crash barbarously into each other, kneeing each other in the stomach or in the first part of the body they are presented with" (Valdés 1792b, 184 [*Mercurio peruano*, 19 July 1792]). Joseph Rossi y Rubí had already discussed the issue a year earlier in his article "Idea de las congregaciones públicas de los negros bozales" [Reflection on the public gatherings of the free blacks], in which he described the very same dance as a series of "ridiculous contortions" incompatible with "the gentleness of our customs," and argued that it was foolish to believe that the actions of blacks "might have the same significance as our own" (Rossi y Rubi 1791, 122). According to Valdés, the physical and moral consequences of these dances would have led blacks to abandon them "if they were not for their most part of an insurmountable stupidity" (Valdés 1792b, 184).

Unfortunately for Pedro Bustamante, he had been suffering from a *bubonocele*, or inguinal hernia, at the time of his death. The repeated jumps and movements of the *Lumbé* aggravated his condition, and at a certain point in the dance "he was violently struck by someone's knee across his herniated tumor, as a result of which his intestine instantly contracted and he was forced to stop dancing because of the violent pain" (ibid., 183–4). He received medical attention at a nearby infirmary, but those who took care of him thought his condition, while serious, was not life-threatening. Valdés came to an entirely different conclusion when he visited the slave the next day. While Pedro had not yet developed a fever, he had spent the night vomiting and complaining of acute pain on the left side of his groin. Valdés considered it likely that Pedro's intestine was pinched or strangulated. Understanding the serious danger his patient was in, Valdés attempted to save him through a dual regimen of bleeding and the administration of oily concoctions and other laxatives, although he conceded that the patient would probably die nonetheless (184). The slave's pain rapidly increased and extended to other parts of his body, and he passed away just thirty-six hours after being hit.

After Pedro's death, Valdés obtained permission to conduct a postmortem examination on the cadaver in order to determine whether the slave's death could have been avoided and to confirm whether he had given the correct diagnosis. After dissecting the abdomen, Valdés found Pedro's punctured intestines "swimming in fecal and pestilent water." The ilium, which "by its position and free movement frequently causes hernias," still showed clear signs of inflammation (185). Valdés inferred from the state of the intestine that Pedro had suffered a double hernia. Therefore, it was not necessary "to be a physiologist or a doctor to understand the indispensable necessity of Pedro's death; regardless of whether the intestine had been violently ruptured by the collision or afterwards by the gangrene, stool had continued to flow in the cavity and had corrupted the intestines." Once the small intestine was broken and separated from the colon, he concluded, death was inevitable. A pessimistic Valdés gloomily informed his readers that "medicine and surgery lack the means of avoiding death in similar situations, and their principles," he concluded, "lead me to affirm that not even in the next centuries will they be found" (188–9).

Valdés's pesimistic predictions about the future of surgery contrasted markedly with Larrinaga's overly optimistic "Disertación de cirugía sobre un aneurisma del labio inferior" [Surgical Dissertation on an Aneurism of the Lower Lip]. Published just three months after his colleague's article, Larrinaga's sought to demonstrate the new levels of sophistication that Lima's surgeons had reached in their art. With feigned humility, he admitted that his essay would probably be of interest only to "a reduced number of readers," but he quickly added that he had no doubt about "the esteem and appreciation with which it would be accepted by his wise and erudite compatriots" (Larrinaga 1792d, 189).

Larrinaga's exposition began with a historical discussion of the causes of various physiological abnormalities and their remedies. He defined an aneurism rather vaguely as "a tumor that forms solely in the arteries and is more or less dangerous, according to the area it occupies, and the causes that produce it," which are often difficult to establish (ibid., 190). For Larrinaga, aneurisms "sometimes occur due to internal causes, such as the lethargy or weakness of an artery, or because of an acrid and corrosive lymph that flows from a near abscess and partially destroys arterial tissue, etc.," while on other occasions "they occur from external causes such as blows, falls, strains, and stings" (190). After reviewing the opinions of Galen, Vesalio, de Haen, and others on the subject, Larrinaga argued that no author, among those who had written on aneurisms and the places where they more commonly occur, had previously described one situated in the mouth or on the lips, or – more importantly – had offered any indication of the appropriate way to operate on such a tumor (195–6). In order to fill this void, Larrinaga offered the readership of the *Mercurio peruano* an account of his own experience with such a case.

Cristóbal González, a Spaniard from Andalusia of about thirty years of age, had consulted Larrinaga about a tumor the size of a dove's egg, which "for about eight years had been growing on the interior part of his lower lip, with neither pain nor change in colour" (197). Cristobal's tumor seemed to have originated from a kick he received from a mule when he was twelve years old (198). Larrinaga examined the lesion and after concluding that it was a true aneurism and not any other kind of deformity or malady, heconsidered the available treatment options. He strongly discouraged Cristóbal from using folk remedies and was particularly averse to "a poultice made from frogs to which he [Cristóbal] had resorted in the past to cure it" (197). As was common when dealing with difficult cases, Larrinaga consulted other surgeons about the best course of action. After taking a vote, they decided that the only feasible option was to operate. Larrinaga's approach was to create a tourniquet using a needle and thread in order to "dry and dissect the artery according to the rules of Velasco and Villaverde" (200).[6] After opening the aneurismal sac with great difficulty, Larrinaga soon ran into problems owing to what he described as an unusual adhesion of its integuments. To solve this unexpected problem, he employed a technique more commonly used to fix cleft lips known as the *pico de liebre* (ibid.; see also Velasco y Villaverde 1763, 380). He then completed the operation by stitching the aneurismal sac in the form of a V and applying the appropriate dressings to the wound (Larrinaga 1792d, 200).

Not everyone agreed with the course of action taken by Larrinaga and his colleagues, and in his article he found it necessary to defend himself against those who had accused him of recklessness because of the great risk of hemorrhage that the operation entailed. He was also criticized for not having used *tenazas aciales* – a special kind of forceps designed for operating on the mouth. Yet, for Larrinaga, the ultimate proof of the suitability of the procedure was that "don Cristobal González today enjoys perfect health without any defect other than those scars caused by the V-shaped incision made with the scalpel in his mouth and the marks left behind by the needles" (212). As for the *tenazas aciales*, he dismissed the accusation by arguing that "the instruments that have been so celebrated in the past century and at the beginning of this one for operating on the *pico de liebre* have been absolutely dismissed by modern surgery as useless and harmful" (210). In this regard, Larrinaga's daring operation illustrates the willingness of eighteenth-century surgeons to try new procedures – frequently risking the lives of their patients – in order to increase their prestige and ensure the continued progress of their art. In a time without general anaesthesia, however, they were often forced to be fast rather than thorough. Surgical complications and postoperative infections caused by poor sanitary conditions meant that many patients died as a result of this kind of intervention (Burke 1977, 34).

Valdés also attempted to enlighten the public about the relevance of the latest scientific theories for the development of surgery. During one of the dissections that took place at the anatomical amphitheatre involving the cadaver of a patient who had died of dysentery, the question was raised whether *aire fijo*, or "fixed air" – as carbon dioxide was commonly referred to at the time – was of any use in the treatment of that illness (Valdés 1793, 87; Woodham 1970, 700).[7] The response to the question was considered interesting at the time not just for its possible benefits for dysenteric patients but also as an illustration of the practical applications of the new chemistry introduced by Jan Baptista van Helmont, Joseph Black, and Henry Cavendish. Valdés addressed the issue in a text that appeared in the *Mercurio peruano* on 10 October 1793.

Valdés did not consider it necessary to describe the specific case discussed at the amphitheatre, since Unanue had already done so in an article that had appeared in the *Mercurio peruano* a few months earlier (Unanue 1793b).[8] He therefore started by describing the forms of dysentery usually observed in Lima and their common remedies, noting that dysentery usually appeared in the fall, especially "if in that season there were repeated alternations between hot and cold weather and if a copious rain failed to purify the atmosphere of humidity and excessive condensation" (Valdés 1793, 89). These conditions reduced transpiration, which in turn stirred and infected the blood through the inertia of the organs that should have purified it. The situation was made worse by the unhealthy dietary habits of many of the city's residents, who ate and drank excessively, leading to "the deprivation of nutrients in the stomach and intestines, the influx of acrimonious bile, and the dissolution of the blood and atrophy of muscles" (ibid.). Individuals suffering from dysentery experienced frequent intestinal pains, nausea and vomiting, runny and serous stool, and "fairly copious amounts of blood in their veins, which dilated because of the irritation." At times, the symptoms were accompanied by fever and chills as well as intense thirst and abdominal swelling.

What really sent many patients suffering from dysentery to their graves was not so much the disease itself but the application of "arcane and empirical remedies" used by many *curanderos* and *viejas,* who confused dysentery with the *enfermedad del vicho* (Valdés 1793, 90; Unanue 1793b, 128).[9] While *curanderos* and *viejas* advised the use of "astringent" remedies in order to contain the dilation of the anus and frequent diarrhea, Valdés – following Unanue – recommended the exact opposite method; he preferred the use of medicines and purgatives that evacuated any feces or putrid fluids.[10] If dysentery was accompanied by intestinal inflammation, the situation could be much more severe. In such cases, Valdés often favoured bleeding the patient and employing antiphlogistic substances instead of laxatives (Valdés 1793, 91–2). Finally, in cases where dysentery degenerated into gangrene, Valdés prescribed the use of antiseptics such as quinine, mixed with lemon juice, and recommended the use of a purgative if there was a sudden interruption in the evacuations; if the appearance of inflammation and gangrene was simultaneous, the prognosis was "decidedly fatal," he noted, "and the devices of the Art have always been frustrated in such circumstances" (93).

It was in such desperate situations that "fixed air" could prove most valuable, since its main property "and the reason for which mankind considers it a useful remedy, is its virtue as an antiseptic, known throughout the learned world" (98). Valdés was referring specifically to the work of Van Helmont, who "realized that meat owes its firmness and consistency to the portion of fixed air it contains and that when meat ferments, it gives off this substance, thereby losing its natural texture and beginning to rot"; he was also referring to the experiments of David MacBride, who supposedly demonstrated the important practical conclusion that "rotten meat can be returned to its original state if one restores the fixed air from which it has been deprived" (Valdés 1793, 98–9). As a result, he maintained, "a piece of rotten meat or fish exposed to the vapour of a material that ferments, [or] to the fixed air that is given off by effervescence, or prepared in such a way that restores the fixed air that it has lost, can avoid decay and be almost entirely recovered" (99). Valdés cautioned that since fixed air had a beneficial effect only on the area where it was applied, its usefulness in the treatment of dysentery was necessarily limited. The irritation of bodily tissues caused by fixed air discouraged its use in the early stages of the illness and also in cases where the patient had "inflammatory" dysentery, since it could increase the inflammation and spasms (101). If gangrene set in, however, there was no remedy as effective as fixed air, since "it corrects the putrid dissolution of fluids much better than other antiseptics and restores firmness to flesh that is already rotten" (ibid.).[11]

According to Valdés, Mr Dehey [William Hey] was the first to experiment successfully with the beneficial effects of fixed air on patients suffering from putrid fever, and this led to the expansion of its application to many other illnesses. As a result, "those suffering from scurvy, cancer, and kidney failure recovered, and the doctors of London and Paris were full of praise for fixed air" (Valdés 1793, 99). On the other hand, there is no indication that Valdés himself ever experimented with its supposed therapeutic virtues. As Woodham has noted, Valdés was untroubled by the fact that "Lavoisier's analysis of the air completely overturned Van Helmont's theories of irreducible elements" (Woodham 1970, 702). The new chemistry only confirmed Valdés's theories on "how to make or where to find carbon dioxide, while an older or less reputable science gave him the basis for his main thesis, that fixed air stops decay" (ibid.). But while Woodham argues that Valdés "completely missed the spirit of the age" by referencing more antiquated findings (ibid.),[12] it could be argued that such "pragmatic" eclecticism was part of the scientific life of Lima at the turn of the nineteenth century. Many doctors in Peru, as in other parts of the Spanish empire, combined the latest scientific theories with others that remained embedded in their medical culture, in spite of having been discredited by some of Europe's leading physicians. In his *Itinéraire descriptif de l'Espagne* (1808), Alexandre Laborde described the teaching of medicine in Spain in 1795 as follows:

Galen's theories were taught in Spanish schools not so long ago. Servile imitators of Galen's verbiage, professors spent almost all their lecture time on useless, annoying, and distasteful things punctuated with barbaric, almost unintelligible jargon and supported by all the subtleties and obscurity of the syllogistic form. It was a flagrant abuse and the consequences were revolting. The Consejo de Castilla recognized the disadvantages and wanted to take the appropriate measures. It ordered professors to limit themselves to explain Boerhaave's *Institutions*. This decree did not have the effect that the government had hoped. Filled with their principles and prejudices, the old professors were allowed to remain. Most of them have circumvented or broken the law. Others have grudgingly complied. They have mixed the Galenic dogmas that they learned as students with the precepts of Boerhaave that have been forced upon them. The resulting combination has created an absurd, unintelligible, monstrous assemblage, a thousand times worse than Galen's doctrine on its own. (Laborde 1809, 5: 178)

While Laborde's opinion conveniently portrayed the backward scientific state of a country that was then at war with France, there is no doubt that physicians in Spain and Peru – as in most parts of the Western world at the time – did not hesitate to combine the most diverse theories as long as they seemed to work and to explain medical phenomena. Two of the fields in which old and new science frequently met were human gender and reproduction.

Gender, Reproduction, and Social Progress

There were few instances when the opinions of surgeons were listened to with more interest in colonial Lima than when discussing issues of sex, gender, and medical monstrosities. The social, religious, and even epistemological confusion that the possibility of hermaphroditism and the crossing of gender boundaries entailed had been the subject of considerable medical, philosophical, and artistic speculation in Spain and colonial Latin America (Burshatin 1998, 3–18; Behrend-Martínez 2005, 1073–93; Horswell 2005, 29–67; Rutter-Jenson 2007, 86–95). Unanue himself had published a note in the *Mercurio peruano* (14 July 1791) entitled "Metamorfoses humanas: Noticias de la extraña desfiguración de una niña" [Human metamorphoses: Report on the strange disfiguration of a girl], in which he affirmed that "there is nothing more natural and common than human transformations" and that "those who consider them to be dreams, visions or fables, have not reflected on the fact that they are not only a real thing, but may even be the origin of the fortune, delight, and instruction of man" (Unanue 1791, 196). At the end of this article, Unanue even provided the address of the unfortunate girl, for those curious enough to see what he was talking about.

Larrinaga addressed this topic in an article he appropriately entitled "En que se trata si una mujer se puede convertir en hombre" [On whether a woman can become a man]. Public interest in the issue had been heightened about a month earlier, when it became known that a nun in Granada had unexpectedly – and inexplicably – developed male genitalia. She had summoned the courage to confess her condition to the archbishop of Granada, Juan Manuel de Moscoso y Peralta, former bishop of Cuzco and Larrinaga's former protector. After a careful physical examination by a surgeon, the ecclesiastic authorities declared her to be a man, and she was subsequently expelled from her convent (Larrinaga 1792b, 230–1).

The role of surgeons in determining the gender of an individual had in fact grown in importance since the seventeenth century as "the Church and State sought to order society through anatomy by identifying manhood through medical examinations instead of depending upon masculine behavior" (Soloudre-LaFrance 2010; see also Behrend-Martínez 2005, 1073; Gorban 2000, 41–55; Few 2007, 159–76). Therefore, as a professor of surgery, Larrinaga considered himself superbly positioned to "satisfy the curiosity of the people of Lima" on the subject and to enlighten readers on the merits of the different theories on gender and sexual difference in use at the end of the eighteenth century (Larrinaga 1792b, 230). He also saw an opportunity to improve his intellectual standing and to demonstrate to those who considered his knowledge "too empirical" that he was "not solely an anatomist," (ibid.).

In an intentional display of erudition, Larrinaga began his article by reminding his readers that such cases were far from unheard-of in classical and contemporary sources. Among them, Larrinaga cited Caeneus's transformation from female to male and back in book 6 of Virgil's *Aeneid*, as well as that of Tiresias in book 3 of Ovid's *Metamorphoses* (Larrinaga 1792b, 231). In the medical literature, Hippocrates himself had described the cases of Phaetusa and Namisia in *Of the epidemics* [*De morbis popularibus*], whose bodies, out of sorrow, became progressively more manly after they had been abandoned by their husbands (233). More contemporary authors such as Juan Fragoso also dealt with the question, specifically addressing the issue of whether a woman could become a man in the fifth question of book 6 of his frequently reprinted *Cirugía universal* (Madrid, 1586), and giving numerous examples of women – many of them nuns – who had become men (see also Vollendorf 2005, 11–31). Following Galen, surgeons such as Ambroise Paré and the aforementioned Juan Fragoso favoured a model in which the male was the dominant gender. According to their theory, women actually had "male genitalia inside their bodies, but this genitalia stayed inside because women had colder bodies than men" (Few 2007, 166). Based on this assumption, it followed that "if women's bodies at some point became unnaturally hot, because of inappropriate work, exercise, and so on, the male genitalia could suddenly emerge, transforming them" (ibid., 167).[13] In opposition to Galen and Paré, those who followed Hippocrates saw sex differences as a continuum, with male and female at its two extremes, leaving the possibility of many positions in between. Finally, those who sided with Aristotle maintained that individuals were "either male or female, with no intermediate possibilities" (ibid.).

For his part, Larrinaga sided with those who defended the mutual irreducibility of the two sexes. He was of the opinion that since sex was a purely anatomical matter, the careful observation of several anatomical characteristics allowed a doctor to distinguish a man from a woman. In the case of men, the most noticeable differences, he argued, were to be found in the perineum, the urethra, and the testicles contained in the scrotum, but he conceded that these characteristics were not always as "obvious and congruent" as they might seem. Some men, for instance, "whom we would call *testicondos*, in keeping with Luchas Scrohlo's work, possess undescended testicles" (Larrinaga 1792b, 234–5). In the case of women, the organ that "should be examined before anything else for the most complete and perfect decision" was the clitoris, "an appendage whose composition is almost entirely the same as the penis except that it lacks the urethra" (235).[14]

Larrinaga also argued that several malformations could complicate correct identification. It was not impossible for the clitoris to be extremely enlarged, as he knew from experience during his time practising in Lima's Hospital de San Bartolomé, where he had examined a clitoris with "a length of nearly six inches." In such extreme cases, he said, there was only one solution: "When such a monstrosity appears, it is necessary to cut it off" (235–6). Yet it was not just the clitoris that

Larrinaga favoured cutting off when it exceeded its usual size. The same went for hypertrophic labia minora that occasionally grew so large that they did not allow patients to walk freely.[15] Thus, Larrinaga advocated a purely "surgical solution" to what he considered a purely anatomical problem. He saw surgeons not only as the "mathematicians" of the flesh defended by Pablo Petit, but also as specialists endowed with the kind of power and expertise necessary to make individuals conform to their "true" nature and ensure that the fundamental difference between male and female remained in place. As for the Granada nun, Larrinaga concluded from his own experiences and without ever having seen the patient that there was absolutely no basis for considering the nun to be a man and much less – as the populace believed – a hermaphrodite (242). She was probably suffering from one of the aforementioned malformations. If anything, her condition was likely to be *un irregular desvío de la naturaleza*, an exceptional deviation from the order of nature, which could have been solved if she had "wanted to suffer secretly the pain of undergoing an almost instantaneous operation from a surgeon" (240).[16]

While the possibility of gender crossing captured the popular imagination, it was the understanding of the mechanics of childbirth and its possible complications that was considered of more immediate practical importance by the doctors and surgeons of the time. Larrinaga addressed the issue in a letter he published on 3 May 1792 with the title "Sobre un fetus de nueve meses que sacó una mujer por el conducto de la orina" [On a nine-month-old fetus born through a woman's urethra]. According to Larrinaga, the case had occurred more than a decade earlier, in 1779, when he was still undergoing training under his mentor, a Spanish surgeon named Francisco Matute. Both were called to examine a girl "who appeared to be fifteen or sixteen years old named Feliciana, or more vulgarly Pichita, who was experiencing strong labour pains, a high fever, nausea, and general weakness two days after repeatedly hitting her abdomen against a door in a fit of passion" (Larrinaga 1792a, 69). After examining the patient, they found that the fetus was clearly situated in the middle of the hypogastrium, but they did not notice any fetal movement. To their amazement, they found the vulva in its natural state but the urethra "extraordinarily dilated," to the point of allowing for the passage of "a foot that slid out with the slightest pull and was still joined to the tibia and the femur" (70). During the following days and weeks, Larrinaga and his mentor continued to extract the fetus's bones through a procedure by which Larrinaga used a catheter to administer "injections of a concoction of quinine, rosebush, and barley, with one ounce of rose syrup, and half an *escrúpulo* [599 mgs] of myrrh dye" in order to prevent infection and facilitate the extraction (70). Such an unusual "birth" did not, however, prevent Feliciana from getting married that same year. Larrinaga reported not having heard from her until three or four years later, when he was called to extract the fetus's last remaining bone – the skull – in an operation that was ultimately carried out by another surgeon, Felipe Bosch (70–1).

To the irritation of some of his colleagues, Larrinaga did not let the opportunity pass to boast about the depth of his knowledge and his powers of observation. He considered that his description of Feliciana's pregnancy surpassed "all the practical knowledge left behind by great thinkers" such as Jean Riolano, Giovanni Domenico Santorini, Jean-Jacques Manget, Paul Bussiere, Guichard Joseph Duverney, and Anelio, all of whom had referenced fetuses found in the Fallopian tubes. In *Zodiacus medico-gallicus* – the Latin version of Nicolas de Blegny's *Nouvelles decouvertes sur toutes les parties de la médecine* (1679) – and in Pierre Dionis there were stories of a number of fetuses that were found in the ovaries; and in the works of Sirausio Baylio, Barthélemy Saviard, Cortial, Joannis Baptistae Bianchi, Alexis Littré, and Raymond Vieussens there were references to fetuses found in the abdomen. None of them, however, gave any indication of how Feliciana's preternatural conception was possible (Larrinaga 1792a, 71–2).[17] According to his own observations, in Feliciana's case there was no perforation or malformation of the uterus, and even the bladder seemed to be completely healthy (74). In fact, she began menstruating sixty days after the procedure. There was also no way to explain how the fetus could have survived so long given that, according to the measurements Larrinaga had taken of its bones, it was already nine months old when it died (82–3). An overconfident Larrianga stated that it was therefore a case without precedent in the medical literature.

The validity of such assertions did not go unchallenged. Many questioned whether a full-term fetus could really develop inside the bladder – as Larrinaga's article seemed to imply – while others dismissed his description altogether. Critics argued that the only way the fetus could have been born as Larrinaga described was if the uterus and the bladder were perforated; and if such was the case, Feliciana should have died from the hemorrhage caused by the internal wounds (76–7). Larrinaga responded to his detractors by reaffirming each and every one of his observations. As for an explanation, he decided to quote Aristotle's *Natura doemonia est* (77).[18] As with the case of the Granada nun, he considered Feliciana's case a deviation from nature. Furthermore, for Larrinaga and others, these types of phenomena, despite being natural occurrences, did not lack religious significance: they were the means through which the divinely inspired order of nature humbled human understanding and reaffirmed the "impenetrable barrier between man and his Creator" (66).

Whereas Larrinaga's interest in gender and reproduction focused on nature's abnormalities, Valdés concentrated on improving the health of pregnant women and training midwives in order to increase childbirth rates and foster population growth. It was an issue in which Unanue was also increasingly interested. As he put it in his "Decadencia y restauración del Perú," it was of the utmost political importance to increase the population of the viceroyalty, since "extensive empires … without inhabitants, are fantastic entities whose magnitude is an imaginary attribute; they are a series of vast solitudes that, far from augmenting the reputation of the Throne, waste its energy" (Unanue 1793a, 87).[19] According to Unanue, pregnancy and childbirth – a realm grossly neglected in the past by public health officials and usually left to priests, women, and charlatans – needed to be treated scientifically and placed in the hands of doctors and surgeons.

Valdés, moved by his "profession, love of country, of science, and of society" (Valdés 1791a, 88), set out to educate mothers and midwives about the most convenient ways of carrying pregnancy to full term in two articles that appeared in the *Mercurio peruano* on 5 June and 25 December 1791.

In the first of these, he said that he considered Lima's mothers to be in great measure responsible for the poor health of their offspring and for their frequent abortions, which he attributed to the ignorance and disorderly appetites of many of them. In his view, most pregnant women in Lima enjoyed a "bland and sedentary life," abused cold drinks and spirits during pregnancy, and continued dancing and bathing without any attention to the consequences of such actions for their unborn children (90). Not surprisingly, many women died during pregnancy, along with their unborn babies, and childbirth thus deprived the country of children who could otherwise have grown up to be "bright torches of the church and knowledgeable in every type of literature" (87). Rather than indulging in those pleasures, Valdés argued, each mother in Lima should concentrate solely on the task of "protecting her fetus, avoiding an abortion, and having a natural birth"; this was greatly facilitated when women were willing to engage in "moderate exercise and a strictly regimented way of life" that allowed them to conserve "their solids and liquids in the necessary equilibrium" (90). Women who remained active, Valdés mantained, did not suffer from fainting spells, their faces were "redder" and their pulse rates much healthier (ibid.). He rejected the opinion of those who considered cravings to be nothing more than a trick that "pregnant women use to satisfy their desires" (90–1). On the contrary, the satisfaction of such cravings, Valdés argued, was of the utmost importance. Depriving the body of the object of its yearning "causes such disorder in its mechanisms that it easily leads to abortion," as evidenced by "the experience of so many unfortunate souls who have perished because of this" (91). Since menstruation stopped during pregnancy, Valdés recommended bleeding pregnant women so that they could eliminate the excess blood retained in their system, although he insisted that the procedure should always be performed under the supervision of an experienced physician, since bloodletting "is often the only safeguard against abortion, but in other cases it may actually facilitate it" (95).[20]

As important as the actions of mothers were for a successful pregnancy, the greatest danger to them and their unborn children was the many charlatans and untrained midwives who usually assisted during labour. The latter were a particular source of concern, since they worked "without any more principles or rules than a blind assistant to the patient and without any more knowledge than that offered by experience itself and the observation of others" (Valdés 1791b, 194). Unanue also considered midwives in Lima to be "women without any ability" who had seized "that delicate part of surgery that is devoted to the care of humanity's offspring: the art of midwifery, an art that requires virtue, quality, and science" (Unanue 1793a, 107). He compared them to a plague, whose "caprice and carelessness have deprived Peru, in countless instances, of the new inhabitants with which nature has charitably sought to compensate for the country's losses, and of the services of fertile mothers who could have helped us forget our misfortune" (ibid.).[21] As a way of remedying the situation and helping midwives avoid the many mistakes they commit during their practice, Valdés sought to provide them with some observations and practical recommendations, based mostly in André Levret's *L'art des accouchements démontré par les principes de physique et de méchanique* (1753), a highly influential book in the emerging field of rational obstetrics (Valdés 1791b, 194; Hibbard 2000, 39).[22]

Following Levret, Valdés saw childbirth as dominated by the invariable laws of physics and hydrostatics. The change in the position of a fetus at the end of gestation was simply the result of the increased weight of its head relative to the rest of its body, while birth resulted from a combination of mechanical forces exerted by both the mother and the infant. Therefore, it was possible to facilitate the process of childbirth by simply understanding its mechanics (Valdés 1791b, 195).[23] For Valdés, women "should be standing, pushing against the ground so that the pressure on the muscles of their feet and thighs is stronger and helps soften [the ligaments of] the pelvis" (197). Once the fetus's head is out, the midwife can help the baby leave the birth canal by carefully pulling with a right-to-left motion. Valdés harshly criticized the practice, common among Lima's midwives, of removing the placenta immediately after birth, which placed women in grave danger of hemorrhaging; he advocated instead that women wait until the body naturally expelled the placenta. He also advised against using "enemas, suppositories, acrid injections, emetics, purgatives" or any other remedies of that kind, which he considered "pernicious and often fatal" and whose use he blamed on the "ignorance of older times and on a less-informed empiricism" (198). Valdés concluded his essay by asking colonial authorities to devote more attention and resources to training midwives correctly, according to enlightened principles. Nevertheless, it was only in the 1820s that a school was created in Lima to that effect.

Incas, Surgeons, and Writers

Both Valdés and Larrinaga considered their contributions, as described in the previous sections, to be more than mere medical curiosities. They judged them to be in line with the journal's ultimate objective of promoting the advancement of their homeland. They wrote their texts and dissertations as "homages" to the fatherland and as a way to "bring glory to Peru" (Larrinaga 1792a, 65; 1792d, 189); or to demonstrate their love of country and "true patriotism" (Valdés 1791a, 87). In so doing, they took ownership of the protonationalist sentiment of the *criollo* elite. This sentiment was already clearly expressed in the first issue of the *Mercurio peruano*. According to editor Calero y Moreira, "the scarcity of information that we have on the country we inhabit and on its interior, and the limited vehicles employed to increase the position of our compatriots in the literary world are the reason why a kingdom such as Peru, so favoured by nature in the goodness of its climate and the opulence of its soil, barely occupies the smallest part in the canvas of the universe as depicted by historians" (Calero y Moreira 1790, 4). He considered the correction of this situation "the founding objective of the *Mercurio*" (ibid.) and added that "what goes on in our nation interests us more than the concerns of a Canadian, Japanese, or Muslim" (ibid., 5).

Valdés and Larrinaga also sought to replicate in their prose the humanistic and erudite style of their colleagues, especially that of Hipólito Unanue. As Woodham points out, Unanue "never considered himself exclusively a physician, and indeed, rarely spoke of himself as such, usually preferring the label 'philosopher,' or more modestly, 'writer' (Woodham 1970, 694). Likewise, Valdés inserted frequent references to classical sources, Latin quotations, and even philosophical and theological reflections in his texts. An example of the latter is found at the beginning of his dissertation on the usefulness of the study of anatomy (1792b). There, he claimed that anatomy was not only useful in understanding the sources of many illnesses and physical problems, but it could even be employed in the fight against one of the most dreaded consequences of the Enlightenment: atheism. Such an "impious sect" would not exist, Valdés argued, if anatomy became a universal study, since there was not a single individual among the unfortunate who belong to that party who could be considered a faithful observer of the structure of the human body. Those who really devoted themselves to the study of anatomy "know God, and by this knowledge, they love Him, resemble Him, and participate in His divine perfection" (ibid., 180).

It was, however, Larrinaga rather than Valdés who more fully explored the possibilities of the *Mercurio peruano* as a means of being seen not just as a surgeon but as a writer and patriot. He did so in two poems in which he addressed one of the fundamental narratives of Peruvian identity: the history of the Inca empire and the transition to Spanish colonial rule. He had been moved to write these poems "not out of ambition for the ephemeral praise usually associated with literary tasks," but in order to "serve [his] beloved country" by singing "the sublime minds that have flourished in this region since the most remote antiquity" (1792c, 17). According to his own words, Larrinaga had hoped that the two poems would also help Peruvian youths better appreciate the history of their fatherland and the civilizing role played by both the Incas and the Spaniards. Or at least that is what he said in 1792 (ibid., 18). Two decades later, already in the midst of the revolutionary wars, Larrinaga revealed in his autobiographical book *Cartas históricas a un amigo* (1812) that he had also intended his poems for the young Prince Ferdinand – the future Ferdinand VII – so that he could learn the history of Peru and the art of ruling an empire (Larrinaga 1812, 161).

Larrinaga's intellectual ambitions were anything but humble. He informed the readership of the *Mercurio peruano* that he had conceived the first poem, on the royal lineage of the Incas, as an introduction to a future book on the history of the Inca empire to be written in imitation of Jean-Baptiste Duchesne's *Compendio histórico de la historia de España*, a French work that had been translated into Spanish by the Jesuit Joseph Francisco de la Isla in 1775 (Larrinaga 1792c, 18). Unfortunately, he had been forced to abandon this project owing to the large amount of time needed "to order the prose that should have accompanied the verses." Nevertheless, he had decided to publish the poem in case other individuals might be willing to perform "this useful service for their country" (ibid.).

Larrinaga's text did not depart significantly from the account the Inca Garcilaso de la Vega had offered almost two hundred years earlier in his *Comentarios reales*. The royal lineage of the Incas had begun with Manco Capac and Mama Coya who, after their appearance on the shores of Lake Titicaca, embarked on a religious and political pilgrimage that culminated with the founding of Cuzco. Larrinaga credited the first Incas, as children of the Sun, for making sure that "the Indians become enlightened / and subjugate themselves with happiness and love." The descendants of Manco Capac and Mama Coya continued their civilizing mission and expanded the empire, thanks to their martial and political skills, as illustrated by the reigns of Sinchi Roca, Inca Roca, and Pachacutec (Larrinaga 1792c, 20–3). The arrival of the Spaniards was already predicted during the reign of the eighth Inca, Viracocha (22). But it was only after the reign of the twelfth Inca, Huayna Capac, that the empire was divided between his two sons, Huascar and Atahualpa, whom he commanded to embrace "with happiness and sincere faith / the laws of other foreign peoples." Unfortunately, Huayna Capac's sons failed to follow their father's orders, and after Atahualpa killed his brother Huascar, the legitimate king, he was deposed and executed by the Spaniards (25).

As for the second poem, devoted to a "chronological succession of the Governors, Presidents, Viceroys, and General Captains who followed the Incas from the conquest to the present," Larrinaga's intent was to demonstrate the legitimacy of the transition to colonial rule, presenting the conquest as a divinely ordered military event and the Spaniards as a people chosen by God to divulge the Gospel and complete the civilizing mission of the Incas (Larrinaga 1793a). Larrinaga placed the blame for the civil wars that followed the fall of the Inca empire on Blasco Núñez Vela, who arrived in Peru in 1544 with the mission of making the conquistadors comply with the New Laws of the Indies. After Nuñez Vela's death at the hands of Gonzalo Pizarro, the mission of restoring peace and order to the colony fell to Pedro de la Gasca, who "entered in the same way as Saint Elmo in the storm, with applause and praise, annulling the cruel ordinances" (Larrinaga 1793a, 163). Larrinaga's "chronological succession" did not go much further. After completing the eulogies of the two viceroys who followed LaGasca – Antonio de Mendoza and the Marquis of Cañete – he ended his poem abruptly, leaving no other explanation than a laconic note in which he stated that "to satisfy those who desire to read this poem, I am publishing the part I have worked on, and so will continue when I have a free moment, because my various occupations do not allow me to do otherwise" (166).

Among the occupations that distracted Larrinaga from writing more poetry was the need to answer a contributor to the *Mercurio peruano* who, under the pseudonym Philaletes, had severely criticized his medical opinions in an article published on 24 February 1793. Philaletes defined himself as "an impartial man who neither thinks systematically nor speaks too passionately" (Philaletes 1793a, 136), even though his only previous contribution to the journal had been a homophobic letter entitled "Carta sobre los maricones" [Letter concerning homosexuals] (Philaletes 1791). To be fair about Philaletes, his criticisms were directed not only against Larrinaga but against several authors whose articles he judged unworthy of having appeared in print. Despite this, much of his text was devoted to questioning not just the findings but especially what he considered the false erudition and heavy literary style of the mulatto surgeon.

Philaletes began by accusing Larrinaga of presumption in claiming that no woman had ever given birth to a fetus through the urethra. To prove his point, he directed Larrinaga to a similar case that had been described in the *Actas de los eruditos de Lipsia*, with a reference to the first German scientific journal, *Acta eruditorum*, founded in Leipzig (Lipsia) by Otto Mencke (Philaletes 1793a, 138). He also found Larrinaga's anatomic disquisition on whether a woman could become a man little more than a sum of "crude and indecent expressions," which should be read only "by those who are in charge of such issues" and not by the public at large (ibid.). He ridiculed Larrinaga's conclusions on the subject, saying that they could have been reached by "any poor peasant" if it were not for the surgeon's extraordinary ability to dress them up "with the verses of Virgil, Ovid, and Langio" (ibid.). Of more substance was Philaletes's questioning of Larrinaga's estimates of the volume of blood in the human body. Larrinaga had addressed this in his article on aneurisms, where he mantained that "a man contains a twentieth part of his body weight in blood and, commonly weighing about 160 pounds, a man will only have about eight pounds of blood" (Larrinaga 1792d, 207). Philaletes offered several alternative estimates calculated by other physicians, such as Quesnai (who put it at 27 pounds) and Hoffmann (28 pounds); he claimed that experience provided numerous examples in which the amount of blood lost by patients well exceeded 8 pounds, and since patients still recovered after having suffered such hemorrhages, he ironically concluded that "they must have remained necessarily with sufficient blood inside their bodies" (Philaletes 1793a, 141).[24] Given the many errors found in his writings, Philaletes said, Larrinaga (whom he mockingly referred to as one of the most "skilful and learned surgeons of our country") should follow the example of Sydenham, Boerhaave, and Haller, who were able to strengthen their reputations further "by confessing their mistakes" (155).

Larrinaga's irate answer appeared on 12 May 1793, signed in his own name, not with his pseudonym. Proving that the use of those pseudonyms was little more than a literary game that he was no longer interested in playing, he remarked that he was well aware of the identity of his critic. He dismissed Philaletes's feigned courtesy simply as rhetoric used to disguise his animosity towards him, and he resented Philaletes's suggestion that he read such books as the *Acta eruditorum*, knowing that he neither possessed nor had the means of acquiring them; moreover, he contended that his critic had intentionally hidden the exact bibliographic reference so that he could not defend himself (Larrinaga 1793b, 28). Philaletes's censure of his article on the Granada nun demonstrated his bad faith even more clearly, Larrinaga noted, adding that even his detractor would accept his conclusions were it not for his desire "to close voluntarily the door of his great understanding in order to question the truth perennially" (ibid., 29). As for the volume of blood in the body and its velocity, Larrinaga pointed out that his calculations exactly replicated those made by Teodoro de Almeida in his *Philosophical Recreations*, and after explaining how this "wise and erudite" doctor had reached his conclusions, he left it to the readers of the *Mercurio peruano* to decide which of the two authors "addresses these subjects briefly and with shameful superficiality, and which one, unsatisfied with such brevity and empty claims, strives to sustain the Truth through solid principles" (Larrinaga 1793b, 31–2; Almeida 1792, 273).[25] Obviously, Larrinaga harboured no doubt about the right answer to his question; but neither did Philaletes.

One month later he answered the challenge in a long letter in which he again refuted each of Larrinaga's arguments and accused the mulatto surgeon of defending his ideas through false erudition and the citation of questionable sources (Philaletes 1793b). Probably fed up with the dispute, Unanue tried to put an end to it and requested that both Larrinaga and Philaletes work together on establishing the usefulness of "fixed air" in the treatment of dysentery, hoping that in doing so they would "omit the hateful controversies that [had] bothered them" (Unanue 1793b, 131). The fact that – as we have seen – it was Valdés who was finally in charge of addressing this subject demonstrates that

Philaletes and Larrinaga were unable to move beyond their mutual hatred. The controversy with Philaletes was, in fact, the first in a series of intellectual confrontations with Lima's medical establishment, and with Hipólito Unanue himself, which put an end to Larrinaga's career, as will be discussed in the next chapter.

While it is true that the mulatto surgeon's medical opinions were self-congratulatory and not scientifically sound, the polemic between Larrinaga and Philaletes indicates a broader problem within the *Mercurio peruano* itself. The scientific value and intellectual originality of the articles had diminished substantially, and its goal of fostering intellectual discussion had given way to petty personal rivalries that undermined the entire project. By 1794, the lack of political and financial support from viceregal authorities meant that the journal was no longer viable, and it ceased publication.[26] Despite its many limitations, however, its contribution to society had been immense. In the few years that elapsed since its first issue, the *Mercurio peruano* had become a foundational reference for those who championed scientific reform and defended the role of modern science – particularly medicine – as a pillar upon which to build the future of the Peruvian viceroyalty and Spanish America. More subtly, the journal also helped to solidify the emerging national consciousness of many creole intellectuals who, in future decades, would help consolidate the independence movement. For Larrinaga and Valdés, it was a public acknowledgement of the high esteem in which they were held as surgeons by Hipólito Unanue and Lima's reformist doctors, in spite of being non-whites.[27] But even more importantly, the *Mercurio peruano* provided Valdés and Larrinaga with the occasion to contribute to the advancement of science and the dissemination of the scientific revolution in Peru while allowing them to establish themselves as writers and public intellectuals at a time when Peru and most of Spanish America were marching towards independence.

CHAPTER 3

Doctors, Citizens, Revolutionaries

In 1806 a royal decree signed by King Charles IV gave Valdés permission to circumvent *casta* regulations and take the required exams to become a doctor. The king's decision came about as a result of the petitions made on Valdés's behalf by a number of influential supporters, including Hipólito Unanue, the Audiencia de Lima, and the city council (Lavalle 1863, 44; Mendiburu 1890, 8: 220). In a sense, it regularized Valdés's irregular professional situation in Lima's medical world. Despite being qualified only as a Latin surgeon, he had received in 1792 temporary authorization to work as a doctor and had been using that prerogative ever since. His biographer, José Antonio Lavalle, points out that a record of this authorization – now lost – still existed in 1858 as part of the archive of the public notary Manuel de Eriza (Lavalle n.d., 4).

Once the royal decree was received in Lima, everything went extraordinarily fast. Before students could obtain a doctorate, university regulations stipulated that they had to obtain their bachelor and licentiate degrees and practise for at least two years under the supervision of a senior physician (*Constituciones y ordenanzas antiguas* 1735, título XI, Constitución xxxiv–xxxvi, xlii–xlix [64v–65r, 66r–68v]). Valdés won every academic degree – the bachelor's, licentiate, and doctorate – in just fifteen days. This was undoubtedly, as Lanning points out, a "plain indication of his impatience to be rid of artificial handicaps" (Lanning 1985, 186–7), but it was also testimony of the power and influence of Valdés's supporters within Lima's medical establishment.

Nonetheless, Valdés's unusually swift passage through all the exams and qualifications of the medical faculty at San Marcos did arouse some animosity.

Surprisingly, the harshest criticism came from his colleague José Manuel Dávalos. Apparently, Dávalos resented the ease with which Valdés had risen from the humble position of Latin surgeon to that of a doctor. He publicly claimed that Valdés had not earned his position on merit but that his good fortune was due to the king's great generosity, "without which for the *zambo* José Manuel Valdés, Latin surgeon of this city, the doors of this university would have been forever closed" (Lavalle n.d. 8; Mendiburu 1890, 8: 220). The racial nature of Dávalos's attack provoked a response from Valdés, who said that "the wedge is good only when it is made of the same wood [as the object it is used to break]," reminding Dávalos that they both shared the same racial origins (Lavalle n.d. 8; Mendiburu 1890, 8: 220).

While Dávalos, Valdés, and Larrinaga did share similar racial origins, this did not mean that they shared the same ideas regarding the future of Peruvian medicine or the same political views. In fact, they did not particularly trust or like each other, as the row between Dávalos and Valdés illustrates. The three of them navigated the treacherous waters of Peruvian medicine and colonial politics separately and with different results. Both Dávalos and Valdés strove to build a reputation and leave their mark for posterity, but without questioning the institutional and scientific paradigm established by Unanue. Of the three, only Larrinaga rebelled against Unanue's authority over Peruvian medicine and against what he saw as the tyranny of the city's predominantly white doctors over its predominantly black surgeons. He paid dearly for it. Race and politics came to the fore in 1812 as the first Spanish constitution opened up for discussion the difficult issue of the political rights of Afro-descendants. The *pardos* and *mulatos* of Lima collectively tried to influence the result of the deliberations by highlighting the critical role they played in the colonial medical world, among other contributions. All hopes were dashed with the return of Ferdinand VII to the throne of Spain in 1814, but the reimposition of the absolute monarchy was not necessarily seen as an evil by everyone. Paradoxically, it was welcomed by Larrinaga, who saw the king as the only person able to rein in the despotism of Lima's doctors and their allies in the viceregal administration. For their part, Valdés and Dávalos adopted a cautious and conciliatory stance. They did nothing to denounce absolute rule in Peru, and they certainly did not join José de San Martín's armies as other blacks and mulattoes did. Nevertheless, when the troops of the Argentine general finally entered Lima in 1821, they both greeted independence with open arms and rapidly commended the new government, in whose administration Hipólito Unanue again played a leading role.

The Anxiety of Influence

Despite his petty remarks about Valdés, Dávalos was no small figure within Lima's medical establishment. He was a fully accredited doctor and a graduate of the University of Montpellier – one of Europe's most prestigious medical faculties – an achievement unmatched by any of his colleagues in the Peruvian capital. His doctoral dissertation, *De morbis nonnullis Limae grassantibus ipsorumque therapeia* [On some common illnesses in Lima and their therapy] (1787), is one of the most important precedents to Unanue's much more influential *Observaciones sobre el clima de Lima y su influencia sobre los seres organizados, en especial el hombre* (1805). Contrary to the argument that American nature and climate contributed to the degeneration of the physical and intellectual abilities of American-born *criollos*, Dávalos maintained that the climate of Lima, like that of Peru in general, was extremely healthy, to the point that it was easy to find many people who lived to be one hundred years old or even older (Dávalos 1787, 4; 7–8). For Dávalos, most illnesses could be traced back to the dietary excesses of the populace, as well as to the pernicious practice of burying the dead inside the city churches (ibid., 10–12; see also Gerbi 2010, 291–2). He nevertheless offered a comprehensive collection of clinical and therapeutical advice for anyone practising medicine in Lima. Each chapter of his book was devoted to a specific malady: paludic fever, cardialgia, cholera, dysentery, hydropsy, cancer, syphilis, scabies, and neonatal seizures (also called in Lima *mal de los siete días*). He was so proud of his work that he believed it had the potential to lead to remedies for "the cruelest maladies that afflict us" (Dávalos 1810, 15). As he put it in his *alegato* to the position of chair of Método de Medicina in 1798,

Gentlemen, I bring you here the insignia of immortality, a work that praises the triumphs of Your Lordship in order to preserve them from the passage of time; a work that contains the remedies for the cruelest maladies that afflict us; a work whose last chapter on the *mal de siete días* is entirely the fruit of my own understanding, since I had no models or documents on which to base my opinions; a work that bears the sweet, glorious, and immortal name of our country on its cover. (Ibid.)

He was not alone. The *Espíritu de los mejores diarios literarios que se publican en Europa*, a journal that collected news published in other European languages for a Spanish readership, observed that Davalos's work had also been favourably reviewed by the editors of the *Journal encyclopédique* (Bouillon, France), who praised the observation skills and erudition of its author (1787, 599).

Yet his path had not been easy. Since he was a mulatto, he had not been able to secure an academic position upon returning to Lima from his medical studies in France. He was even accused of plagiarizing his doctoral thesis, and he had to take his medical exams again (Lastres 1955, 158). After working as a professor of chemistry for one year, he was offered the chair in Botany in 1796, only to be relieved of it shortly afterwards in favour of the Spaniard Juan Tafalla. In 1798 he presented himself to the position of chair of Método de Medicina, which was eventually awarded to Miguel Tafur (ibid., 159–60). Despite all these setbacks, Dávalos was able to establish a solid scientific and intellectual reputation in Lima. In 1806, the same year that Valdés became a doctor, Viceroy Abascal designated Dávalos as substitute chair of Vísperas de Medicina, the second most important position in the university curriculum after the chair of Prima de Medicina. For his part, Unanue, who in 1794 had invited him to lecture at the anatomical amphitheatre, offered him a faculty position in his future Colegio de medicina y cirugía de San Fernando (ibid., 1955, 161; Dejo Bustios 2008, 217). Also in 1806, Dávalos – and not Valdés – was granted the honour of playing a leading role in one of the most ambitious public health efforts ever attempted by the Spanish Crown: the smallpox vaccination campaigns.

Five years after Edward Jenner published his observations and experiments on the cowpox virus, King Charles IV mandated that an expedition be organized with the purpose of taking the vaccine to every corner of the Spanish empire. Under the direction of royal court physician Francisco Javier de Balmis, the Real Expedición filantrópica de la vacuna, as it was known, departed from La Coruña on 30 November 1803. It carried twenty-two orphan children, who were inoculated with the vaccine during the trip in order to maintain the strength of the vaccine lymph and allow for arm-to-arm vaccinations once the expedition reached the Americas (Lanning 1940, 124; Mark 2009). Upon arrival, the expedition divided into two groups, with Balmis leading a campaign to Cuba, Mexico, and the Philippines while José Salvany, a Spanish surgeon, performed vaccinations in Colombia and Peru. After a hazardous and eventful journey through the Andes that almost cost him his life, Salvany arrived in Lima on 23 May 1806. If he expected a hero's welcome in the Peruvian capital, he was disappointed. Vaccines had already reached Lima from Buenos Aires, the capital of the viceroyalty of Río de la Plata, having arrived there in August 1804 from samples sent to Brazil via Portugal (Mark 2009, 83). By the time Salvany set foot in Peru, Lima's physicians were fully aware of Jenner's work. They had even experimented with vaccination procedures and carried out their own immunization campaigns (Lanning 1940, 123). Even worse, many doctors regarded Salvany as an outsider who knew nothing about Peru and the country's diseases, and they were quick to dismiss his ideas (Warren 2010, 105).

In compliance with royal instructions, however, Viceroy Marquis de Avilés asked Salvany to enact his plan to carry out the vaccination campaign and establish a committee charged with overseeing the conservation and distribution of the vaccine. The Audiencia de Lima then appointed Salvany director of the Junta central para la preservación y propagación de la Vacuna (Central Committee for the Preservation and Propagation of the Vaccine), and named as its medical consultants José Manuel Dávalos and Pedro Belomo, a Spanish surgeon who had been responsible for bringing the vaccine from Buenos Aires and was also the first to perform smallpox vaccinations in Lima using Jenner's technique. (Warren 2010, 78–9, 107).[1] It did not take long for tensions to surface. In fact, the relationship with Salvany deteriorated so rapidly that by September 1806, the city council had proposed that the direction of the vaccination campaign be placed in the hands of Dávalos and Belomo. Salvany bitterly protested that he had been appointed by the king to lead the campaign and criticized the lack of support offered by

Lima's civil authorities. He also accused his colleagues – especially Dávalos – of being preoccupied with their own social advancement rather than with the health of their patients, and claimed that they had failed to take the necessary steps to ensure the success of vaccinations throughout Peru. Dávalos and Belomo dismissed Salvany's criticisms and replied that together they had already saved eight thousand lives from smallpox before Salvany's arrival in Lima (ibid., 110). In the end, Salvany's resistance proved futile. In early 1807 he was forced to hand over three of the children under his care that had recently developed pustules as result of vaccination. He left the city soon afterwards to continue his vaccination campaigns in Arequipa and other parts of Peru before dying in Cochabamba in 1810 (ibid., 111).

Meanwhile, vaccinations in Lima progressed far less smoothly than anticipated. Many residents refused to participate or allow their children to be vaccinated after a rumour spread that the vaccine was not only ineffective but might be dangerous. In order to quell popular resistance, Dávalos decided to take the campaign to the "streets, plazas, suburbs, and other notable places" instead of waiting in designated areas for prospective patients to appear – he later complained about the distrust with which many viewed his work, believing "that the vaccine is an evil and not an antidote" (Dávalos 1818, 494). Dávalos and his assistants even considered coercing caregivers to vaccinate their children and babies, but since they lacked the authority and means to do so, they were forced to devote a substantial amount of their time to "persuading, begging, and rewarding mothers so that, for the good of their children, they would allow them to be vaccinated" (495). He was also particularly troubled by the worsening quality of the pustules from which the vaccine was extracted, which he blamed on epidemics and other unforeseen circumstances beyond his control (495–6). Despite this and other setbacks, the campaign was, by most measures, an unqualified success, and Dávalos continued lobbying the authorities for financial and material resources until his death in 1821, when his position was offered to none other than José Manuel Valdés (Gamio Palacios 2005, 294 [Sesión de Cabildo de 30 de octubre de 1821]).

Professional rivalries may have played an important role in fuelling Davalos's animosity towards Valdés. Valdés had been at the centre of medical discussions in Lima before Dávalos's return to Peru. Thus, while Dávalos had to build his reputation in the city after his arrival, Valdés had enjoyed from the very beginning the support and recognition from Unanue and his colleagues, who invited him to lecture at the anatomical amphitheatre and publish his ideas in the *Mercurio peruano*. Even worse, while Dávalos – as a graduate from Montpellier – had to fight to have his degree fully recognized in order to practise medicine, Valdés – a Latin surgeon – was being granted privileges reserved for doctors. Things did not stop there. As his prestige grew, an emboldened Valdés began to offer his opinions more and more often on medical subjects, some of which Dávalos considered he had already adequately addressed in his *De morbis nonnullis Limae grassantibus ipsorumque therapeia* (1787). This was the case with the neonatal seizures known as *mal de los siete días*, which Dávalos had addressed in his dissertation and for which Valdés recommended the use of copaiba balsam (Dávalos 1787, 111–35; Valdés 1815a).

Valdés first publicly presented his experiences with copaiba balsam during his medical exams, although he did not publish his findings until 1815 when they were included as part of his *Disertaciones médico-quirúrgicas* (1815a, 5). The anti-inflammatory properties of copaiba balsam – an oleoresin also known as Jesuit's balsam and *palo de aceite* – were well known, but its use in the treatment of neonatal seizures was a relatively novel idea. In 1795 a royal decree had recommended that the navels of infants be anointed with balsam to avoid epilepsy and convulsions (Lanning 1940, 125). Valdés accused many doctors in Lima of ignoring this advice and treating the seizures with nothing more than "Greek gibberish that does not mean what they had intended" (Valdés 1815a, 29–31). Whether this was a veiled reference to Dávalos is unclear, but he was not alone in considering the issue far from settled. Unanue himself lamented that many mothers, because of the lack of appropriate medical advice, made the fatal decision to turn to unlicensed medical practicioners when their children experienced such convulsions:

> The mother is absorbed in contemplation of the infant in her lap, who has been surprised by an unexpected tremor. His eyes are already closed, flashing and quivering, his limbs contracting and lengthening with violent and alternating agitation, upsetting the pleasant visage of innocence, and his discordant voice announcing in sad cries the fatal poison that devours him; she holds him

in her arms, showering the child with her tears, puts him down, and runs with terror in search of help. But alas! Instead of help, she only finds barbaric hands that sacrifice her child! (Unanue 1793a, 95)

Valdés's description of the symptoms was no less vivid and was written in a very similar tone:

The tender child moans oppressed by anguish, and a series of extraordinary movements occur throughout his entire body; his eyes now remain fixed and now rapidly rotate and turn around; and with dilations and contractions, his limbs become twisted and then disentangle. The restless movements of the unhappy Laocoön were not any greater when he attempted to free himself from those two atrocious serpents that, eating his flesh and coiled tightly around his body, were putting an end to his movements and to his life while their horrific and bloodied heads towered over his shoulders. I shudder at the thought of it! (Valdés 1815a, 19)

In Valdés's view, the condition was linked to an underlying digestive problem caused by several factors, the chief being Lima's climate. According to him, the heat and humidity caused the city's inhabitants to suffer from a weak physical constitution, which predisposed them to convulsive illnesses as a result of inadequate digestion (Valdés 1815a, 35). In such an environment, food easily spoiled in the stomach, which caused convulsions as the body attempted to expel it. In the case of breastfed children, the situation was often aggravated by their mother's milk turning sour, resulting in "a bitter serum that stimulates and damages the lining of the stomach" (37). Strong emotions, especially anger, also had the potential to corrupt the milk of nursing mothers, which in turn could result in convulsions leading to the infant's death. In such cases, Valdés argued, the only possible remedy – far superior to the traditional methods, which included baths, opium, and cascarilla – was to give suffering children from one *escrúpulo* to half a *dracma* [1 *dracma* = 3 *escrúpulos* = 3.5944 grams] of copaiba balsam as soon as the convulsions started (25). He based its effectiveness on the balsam's ability to "expel diverse materials from the body that are found in the abdomen and simultaneously give greater tone to the body's organs so that they are less sensitive to peculiar stimulants and can more easily digest food" (39). He assured his readers that by following this method, "the good God has allowed me to save hundreds of children from the danger they were in," and he insisted that the medicinal virtues of the balsam were such that convulsions "frequently stop right after the first dose" (25–7).

In his attempt to build up his reputation as a physician, Valdés was willing to take certain risks, challenge the conventional wisdom held by his colleagues, and even scandalize Lima's rather conservative upper class. This is illustrated by his approach to uterine cancer, which Dávalos had also addressed in his *De morbis nonnullis Limae grassantibus ipsorumque therapeia* (1787, 87–94). Valdés presented his ideas on the issue at a conference held in the anatomical amphitheatre in 1801, where he questioned the medical consensus that uterine cancer was highly contagious (Valdés 1815, 1).[2] To the outrage of many of his compatriots, who strongly condemned him for exposing to public scrutiny "maladies that have generally remained hidden and are embarrassing for their kind," he gave as an example the case of a woman from Lima's upper class who had died of uterine cancer a year earlier (Lavalle n.d., 6–7). The woman in question was Carmen Bravo de Lagunas, wife of Tomás Muñoz y Lobatón, Marquis of Casa Muñoz. After Carmen's death, her family followed the customary procedures for dealing with the property of those who had died of an infectious disease, regardless of whether the victim was rich or poor. In order to avoid contagion, "they threw all the furniture and objects that had been directly used by the deceased into a fire; they placed her finest clothing and most precious jewels on statues of the Virgin and of saints, distributing the less valuable items amongst servants and beggars; and they stripped the walls and changed the upholstery and tiling throughout the house" (Lavalle n.d., 6). In Valdés's opinion, such practices were the result of pure ignorance. Uterine cancer, he argued, does not pre-exist or cause the ulcer, as it would if it were an infectious disease; rather, the ulcer itself becomes carcinogenic as a result of improper care and the degeneration of the surrounding tissue (Valdés 1815c, 104–5, fn).

Valdés attributed the frequency of the disease in Lima to a combination of factors: the weakness of its inhabitants' blood vessels, which he considered a consequence of the capital's proximity to the Pacific Ocean; the putrid miasmas emanating from the many crypts that existed in the city; and the sedentary lifestyle of Lima's female residents.

Since the uterus contains a large number of blood vessels, Valdés reasoned, it is only natural that it is more susceptible to cancer than other organs (Valdés 1815c, 111). According to Valdés, "social maladies" also contributed to the high incidence of the disease. Abortions and undesired pregnancies were common in the Peruvian capital, particularly among lower-class women, and there was also a harmful tendency among women of all social standings to "conceal their pregnancies" through the use of girdles and tight clothes that often damaged the uterus (116–17). Finally, charlatans, folk healers, and untrained surgeons helped "propagate." uterine cancer through their waters, powders, and inadequate interventions, which frequently made the most benign ulcers cancerous (120–1, fn). Regardless of the cause of the malady, Valdés argued, since there was no risk of contagion, it made no sense to quarantine patients and destroy their personal belongings. Even if transmission were possible, the only measures necessary to prevent the spread of infection would be "fresh air and water, or mixtures containing aromatics, and antiseptics [that] completely purify the furniture, even those that have been used by the patients" (113–15, fn). As Valdés probably expected, his claims about uterine cancer were hotly challenged by his peers in Lima. Yet the controversy did little harm to his career. On the contrary, it helped solidify his reputation in the capital as one of the most daring and sophisticated physicians of his age. His prestige grew when it became known some years later that Françoise-Emmanuel Foderé had made the same arguments in his influential *Traité de médicine-légale et d'hygiène publique ou de police de santé* (1813 [1798], 1: 349; Valdés 1838, 15n4]).

The professional rivalry between Valdés and Dávalos was to a certain extent settled when Unanue offered both of them faculty positions at his proposed Colegio de medicina y cirugía de San Fernando. Backed by Viceroy José Fernando de Abascal y Sousa, work on the school's construction began in June 1808. It was to be centrally situated on the Plazoleta de Santa Ana, adjacent to the Hospital of San Andrés and close to the major hospitals of Santa Ana, San Bartolomé, and La Caridad, as well as the old botanical garden. Strongly influenced by the ideas of Herman Boerhaave and the intellectual tradition associated with the Leiden School, Unanue decided to dispense with the traditional structure that had regulated the teaching of medicine at San Marcos since the seventeenth century. He proposed a curriculum of eighteen subjects that would be divided into four main branches: medicine, mathematics, physics, and natural history (Unanue 1808). Medicine would in turn be divided into two fields: theoretical medicine – comprising zoonomy, pathology, and psychology – and practical medicine – composed of clinical medicine, surgery, obstetrics, pharmacy, and topography. The objective was not simply to educate future physicians but also to develop enlightened scientists, versed as much in medicine and surgery as in the sciences that Unanue considered key for a proper understanding of the profession. In addition to students residing in Lima, the school would open its doors to them coming from other parts of Peru through a grant program funded by the provincial authorities.[3] Unanue expected that, upon graduation, these students would return to their home regions and help extend modern science and medicine to every corner of Peru, thus achieving a goal he had first envisioned at the opening of the anatomical amphitheatre more than a decade earlier. To this end, he was able to recruit some of Lima's most prominent physicians as faculty members. Dávalos, who in 1809 had been given the interim position of chair of Vísperas de Medicina at San Marcos, became chair of Materia Médica at the Colegio de San Fernando (Lastres 1955, 161). As for Valdés, he was named examiner in Surgery and chair of Clinical Medicine in 1811 (Lavalle n.d., 15; Mendiburu 1890, 8: 221; Romero 1942, 305). Of the three most distinguished mulatto surgeons and physicians of their time, Larrinaga was the only one to be excluded from this project, upon which Unanue had placed much of his hopes for the reform of medicine in Peru.[4]

A Surgeon's Demise

After the publication of Larrinaga's *Apología de los cirujanos del Perú* in 1791 and his contributions to the *Mercurio peruano* in 1792 and 1793, his attention shifted to the commendable project of creating a fund to relieve the many "miseries and misfortunes" to which the families of elderly and deceased surgeons were frequently subjected after a life of service (*Ordenanzas de la sociedad patriótica del monte pío de los cirujanos del Perú* 1802, 2).[5] The Sociedad patriótica del Monte Pío de los cirujanos del Perú, as the fund was called, was formed following the example of similar institutions created in Spain for the support of military personnel (Rabí Chara 2001, 113). The surgeons of the city unanimously approved its governance structure and operating rules on 13 May 1799. One year later, Viceroy Ambrosio O'Higgins, Marquis of Osorno, ratified them pending final approval from Madrid. The municipal magistrate Tiburcio de Mendoza y Ríos was in charge of sending the documents on behalf of Larrinaga and his colleagues, and in 1802 he asked the king to approve their request "in spite of being all of them *pardos*," on account of their many servicies, their "irreproachable conduct," "elegant manners," and the "wisdom they demonstarted in their procedures" (AGI, Lima 1010, Memorial de José Pastor de Larrinaga, letter sent by Tiburcio de Mendoza y Ríos on 24 December 1802, document 9). To the satisfaction of those involved, Charles IV did so by a royal decree dated 23 July 1803.

Larrinaga saw the constitution of the Sociedad patriótica as only a first step in a much more ambitious and controversial institutional agenda. His plan was to dissociate the – mostly black – city surgeons from the supervision of the Protomedicato and the – mostly white – doctors who dominated it. This did not take long to occur. Already, on 5 April 1801, Charles IV had ordered the creation of the Junta superior gubernativa de los reales colegios de cirujía and ordered that the study of medicine and surgery be done separately. Three years later, on 2 March 1804, the king explicitly banned his protomédicos in America from "direct and indirect knowledge of everything concerning surgery" and ordered that *Juntas gubernativas de cirujía* and surgical schools be created in the Spanish dominions for the certification and control of colonial surgeons (Rabí Chara 2001, 106–8). This was a dream that Larrinaga had long nurtured. Tiburcio de Mendoza y Rios's letter requesting the creation of the *Sociedad patriótica* had emphasized the convenience of creating such a school in Lima "in immitation of those in Spain" so that the city surgeons could demonstrate "their high level of education and their skill in the art of healing" (AGI, Lima 1010, Memorial de José Pastor de Larrinaga.).

In 1805, in line with the king's wishes, Larrinaga presented the viceregal authorities with his plans for the creation of a school of surgery. It was to be located at the Hospital of Saint Bartolomé and named Colegio de cirugía de San Carlos in honour of Charles IV. The proposal included the creation of a *Junta de cirugía* to supervise the school and everything connected with the certification and control of the city's surgeons. This body was to be formed by Ramón Castro, Bernardo

Acevedo, Hipólito Lizárraga, and Larrinaga himself as the current pro-tocirujano (surgeon examiner) at the Protomedicato. For the school's faculty members, Larrinaga mentioned the names of José Santos Montero, Francisco Faustos, and Manuel Cáceres, among others, but tellingly not José Manuel Valdés, even though he was still a Latin sur-geon. To help establish the new institution – in which students would learn anatomy, chemistry, and botany as well as surgery – all faculty members, including Larrinaga, offered to teach free of charge and even to donate the instruments and books necessary for the students' in-struction until the school could be appropriately funded through other sources. With it, Larrinaga hoped to demonstrate that he and the thirty surgeons who had granted him power of attorney were moved not by ambition for "glory or titles" but by the desire to remedy "the death of hundreds of Indians, delegates, priests, merchants, and miners" who frequently died from their wounds owing to the lack of properly edu-cated surgeons (AGI, Lima 1010, Memorial de José Pastor de Larrinaga, Instrucción al apoderado de Madrid con arreglo al poder que le han conferido a su protocirujano los profesores de cirugía, 26 June 1806).

Larrinaga's proposal was received with animosity by the current protomédico, Juan José de Aguirre, and especially by Hipólito Unanue, who at the time was planning the future Colegio de medicina y cirugía de San Fernando. Unanue was charged by the viceregal authorities with the task of evaluating the proposal, and Larrinaga accused him of writ-ing "a libelous report, a draft of which was widely circulated before being presented to the authorities" in which Unanue ridiculed the whole project (AGI, Lima 1010, Memorial de José Pastor de Larrianga, letter dated 7 August 1808, document 4). Larrinaga demanded to have access to Unanue's report, citing "the fair, necessary, and precise obli-gation to defend his opinions and good name, dispelling completely the false, ridiculous, and untimely accusations that had been levied by his colleagues in that text." But it was to no avail (ibid.). In view of the contempt and silence of the Peruvian authorities, he decided to appeal his case directly to the king, and shortly afterwards he sent his pro-posal to Madrid. He included the powers of attorney of twenty city surgeons and complained that Unanue and Viceroy Abascal "have managed to convince some of them to withdraw it with false argu-ments" in order to prevent "the necessary establishment of a school of surgery" (AGI, Lima 1010, letter of José Pastor de Larrinaga, 8 August

1808). Unfortunately for Larrinaga, the French invasion of the Iberian Peninsula got in his way. A year later, Larrinaga again complained about the silence of the viceregal authorities with regard to his request and expressed his bewilderment at not knowing, as a result of the war, if his proposal had been received in Madrid and whether it had been approved by the king.

Larrinaga's adversaries reacted swiftly. In 1807 Viceroy Abascal approved Unanue's project for the Colegio de medicina y cirugía de San Fernando, whose construction started one year later, even though it lacked official approval from Madrid. That same year, Larrinaga lost his position as protocirujano at the Protomedicato in favour of one of his detested "overseas surgeons," the Spaniard Pedro Belomo, who had been chosen over him in 1806 to carry out the smallpox vaccination campaigns together with Salvany and Dávalos (Rabí Chara 2006b, 24). Of more consequence to his economic situation, Larrinaga was removed by order of the viceroy from his position as surgeon of the military unit, Regimiento de dragones de Carabayllo, a post he had held since 1780. Another mulatto surgeon, Pedro de Utrilla, a descendant of the famous family of seventeenth-century surgeons portrayed in Caviedes's *Diente del Parnaso*, was appointed to replace him. Larrinaga complained bitterly to colonial and metropolitan authorities about the abuses he endured. In 1809, he once again wrote to the king asking him to overturn the decisions taken by Viceroy Abascal and the protomédicos Juan José de Aguirre and Hipólito Unanue, imploring his protection from the threats and false accusations that the doctors of Lima had made against him and other surgeons in order to "despotically control the Faculty of Medicine" (AGI, Lima 1010, Memorial de José Pastor de Larrinaga, Demanda de satisfacción de los daños y perjuicios que le han ocasionado en su fama, honra y hacienda los protomédicos del Perú).

Unanue and those who, like Dávalos and Valdés, formed part of his intellectual circle sought not only to isolate Larrinaga institutionally and professionally but also to destroy his scientific reputation. The occasion to do so emerged with the publication of Larrinaga's observations about the fetus aborted by an African slave, which appeared in a special supplement of the *Gaceta de Lima* on 28 April 1804. He later recounted the circumstances of the abortion and the events that followed it in his book *Cartas históricas a un amigo* (1812), a defence of

his professional standing and a condemnation of Lima's most distinguished doctors, including Unanue, Valdés, and Dávalos.

The episode had taken place in the outskirts of Lima three weeks
earlier, on 6 April 1804. That morning, the slave overseer Cristobal
Castañeda found a pregnant slave named Asunción suffering in her bed
from excruciating pain in her lower abdomen and experiencing moderate vaginal bleeding. Castañeda then sent word to the Marquis of
Fuentermosa, Asunción's owner, so that he could make the appropriate decision about how to proceed:

> After learning about the events in his *chácara* [small estate], and
> demonstrating the piety that is such a defining characteristic of
> him and his family, the marquis immediately sent his carriage
> for a midwife of high intelligence and good character named
> Mercedes Ramírez who, in the company of Cayetana Gómez,
> one of his servants, was ordered to help the negra Asunción and
> to spare no expense. They were also told to treat the slave in
> the *chácara* if her condition allowed it or to take her to Lima,
> observing all the precautions that the risk of a miscarriage de-
> manded. They arrived there ... at half past two in the afternoon
> and found the woman losing a great amount of blood, com-
> plaining of sharp pain in her hips and waist, and with the head
> already crowning. After examining it with her fingers and feeling
> something like a spine, the midwife thought that the skull might
> be fractured. She then gave the slave a hearty soup to help her
> gather strength and encouraged her to push even harder. After
> this, with the help of the aforementioned Mercedes Ramírez,
> Asunción expelled from her womb a young pigeon. (Larrinaga
> 1812, 2–3)

In the midst of considerable confusion, the midwife and the house-
maid decided to take Asunción to Lima, where Larrinaga was called to
attend to the patient. He then performed an examination on the slave
and dissected her fetus in front of the wife of the Marquis of Fuente-
hermosa and other members of her family and service. Upon finishing
the procedure, Larrinaga concluded that Asunción displayed all the
symptoms of having suffered a miscarriage and that her fetus had
indeed the "body and figure of a pigeon with a length of two inches and

six lines from the spine's first vertebrae to the tailbone and that it lacked a head, a neck, wings, and feet" (3–5). He decided to leave the corpse inside a glass container filled with alcohol "so that the house physician, Dr Miguel Tafur, and those who so desired could examine it with their own eyes" (5). Larrinaga examined Asunción once again later in the day in order to ensure that the patient was stable, having suffered such an unusual miscarriage, and he was then surprised to find in her belly a bump that the midwife incorrectly believed to be the afterbirth; after realizing that it was a body, which moved at the slightest touch, he concluded that Asunción remained pregnant, with another three- or four-month-old fetus (ibid.). Larrinaga pointed out that it was necessary to wait and avoid making any assumptions about what remained in Asunción's womb until it had been delivered: "We cannot know *a priori* if at seven or eight months she will give birth to a *mola* [a disfigured fetus] or, if at nine months, which is the ordinary term, a human being; or if it will be some other extraordinary phenomenon like the one we have in front of us" (7).

That the case of a slave interested an educated surgeon such as Larrinaga was less extraordinary than it might seem. Asunción was a black woman who worked outside the city in miserable living arrangements, the type that often led to life-threatening illnesses and rare medical conditions. Unanue himself considered increasing the rate of succesful childbirths and improving the health of those at the bottom of society as key to the long-term prosperity of the viceroyalty (1793a). Larrinaga may also have been motivated by the impulse to provide a first-hand account of the birth of a "monster." Many other doctors and writers in Lima – including Unanue – had mused about the possibility of deformed and animal-like creatures being born to humans, and their descriptions, rather than being rejected, had found a place in journals such as the *Mercurio peruano*.[6] For his part, Larrinaga based his defence on the numerous treatises on monstruosities still widely read at the time.[7] Already in his article for the *Gaceta de Lima*, he had anticipated the need to defend his observations and thus offered the public what he considered to be relevant precedents to Asunción's monster:

Amidst all the happiness given by the heavens to Robert King of France in the eleventh century, he had the misfortune of seeing Queen Constance give birth to a monster with the head and neck of a gosling ... and the rest of its limbs corresponding to those of a human, as explained by Saint Pedro Damiano, Archbishop of Ravena. Even in our own Spain, the celebrated Luis Mercado [personal doctor to Felipe II and Felipe III] saw a noblewoman who had been sterile for fifteen years give birth to three *molas* [a desfigured fetus] after three successive pregnancies, and in the fourth one she gave birth to a monster that had deformed eyes, lacked nostrils, and possessed a mouth and lips like the beak of an eagle. (Larrinaga 1812, 3–4)

Given these and other examples provided in the aforementioned works, Larrinaga concluded that it was entirely possible that a human body might produce a fetus that did not resemble a human being. Far from being forbidden by natural law, the birth of such monsters proved that God and nature had the power to disobey and "deviate" from their own rules where and whenever they saw fit (125).[8]

Even with these recent precedents, Larrinaga's article was fiercely contested, despite the fact that he had conceded in his essay that he did not have the slightest idea how a bird could have grown inside a human uterus (Larrinaga 1812, 7). Yet the mere suggestion that a woman could conceive a young pigeon was enough to elicit the cruelest of criticisms from the doctors of Lima, who were of the opinion that Larrinaga's description openly contradicted the theories of human reproduction that were considered valid at the beginning of the nineteenth century. The most compassionate of his detractors sought a "rational" alternative explanation for what had happened to the black slave. One harsher critic advanced the hypothesis that "Asunción could have inserted a pigeon's egg on a whim in order to incubate it in her privates" (ibid., 8–9). Whether the hypothesis was intended as a joke is uncertain, but Larrinaga certainly did not take it as one. He refuted his critics by arguing that the monster's birth was preceded by all the symptoms expected in a true miscarriage, including pain in the lower abdomen and hemorrhaging. As for the idea that she might have incubated an egg, he asked his opponents, "How could the internal orifice of the uterus have widened if this pigeon's egg had been fertilized lower down – that is, inside the vagina – as was the opinion of the author of the pointed argument we have just seen put forward" (ibid., 9).

In an attempt to settle the issue and put an end to any further arguments, José Manuel Dávalos invited Larrinaga, Tafur, Unanue, and Valdés to a series of meetings aimed at finding the truth. They were supposed to meet with open minds and without any prejudice against Larrinaga, but it soon became clear that Dávalos's intention was to prove that the young pigeon could not have been born to Asunción and had most likely been placed in her vagina before the "miscarriage." Some argued that Asunción "may have placed the young bird in her vagina for ends motivated by her maliciousness or because it was all a form of witchcraft" and that civil and eclessiastical authorities would have a word or two to say about the matter (Larrinaga 1812, 36). Dávalos' own anatomical dissection of the "fetus" revealed, he claimed, the existence of seeds of wheat and mustard in the monster's intestines, which proved beyond doubt that it was an animal that had formed outside Asunción's body. For Larrinaga, however, the fact that Davalos's examination had taken place without his authorization and without him being present raised the suspicion that Dávalos might have placed the seeds inside the monster's body in order to prove his argument. Larrinaga responded by questioning how it was possible to find the seeds in such a good state of conservation inside the animal's intestines more than thirty days after having its birth. He also challenged Dávalos to explain how it was possible for the presumed animal to have eaten those seeds if, according to Dávalos's own anatomical examination, it lacked a neck. Confronted with these arguments, those present at the meeting maintained a guilty silence, noted Larrinaga, "and, at that point, my friend, they all seemed much more suspicious of me" (ibid., 26).[9] Larrinaga had finally understood that despite sharing the same racial origins, Valdés and Dávalos had sided with Unanue and left him completely alone.

Medicine and Citizenship

Political events in the Iberian Peninsula conspired to bring the three black physicians together in pursuit of a common goal, at least temporarily. The war with France and the convocation of the Cortes de Cádiz in 1810 culminated in the proclamation of the Spanish Constitution of 1812. Among the most contentious issues discussed during the constitutional debates was the question of who should have the right to full Spanish citizenship and, with it, the right to vote in local and parliamentary elections. According to the imperfect population estimates used in Cadiz at the time, if all those living in the New World were granted the right to full citizenship, the balance of voting power would shift to the Americas, thus making Spain a *de facto* colony within its own empire. Such an outcome was unacceptable for many metropolitan representatives, who sought to exclude large sections of the population – especially *castas* and those of African ancestry – from direct political representation.[10] Nevertheless, not everybody shared such a restrictive view of citizenship rights. Some American representatives argued that by not granting full citizenship to all those who were born in Spanish America, the Cortes risked fanning the flames of rebellion and encouraging the spread of the insurrections that had started in the viceroyalties of Nueva Granada and Rio de la Plata (King 1953a, 34). Proponents of broader citizenship rights also emphasized the substantial contributions made by the lower castes to the survival and prosperity of the colonies (Morán Ramos 2010, 117). The polemical issue was finally debated between 4 and 7 September 1811 for inclusion in the Cádiz Constitution as Article 22 (*Diario de las discusiones y actas de las Cortes* VIII, 4 de septiembre–7 de septiembre de 1811, 143–225). The final wording of the article established that Spanish citizenship was to be granted to those individuals of African descent who "perform qualified services for their country or are distinguished by their talent, application, and conduct, with the condition that they be of legitimate birth; that they be married to a woman of good standing and settled in the dominions of Spain; and that they work in a useful profession, office, or industry with their own capital" (*Constitución política de la monarquía española* 1820 [1812], 9–10, art. 22). While the article seemed to open the door of citizenship to individuals of African ancestry, in practice it made it almost impossible for them to obtain, given their general lack of economic resources, the high number of illegitimate births in that segment of the population, and the existing restrictions against Afro-Peruvians in the educational system and most professional guilds.

Unsurprisingly, the conditions set out in Article 22 were met with indignation by the many blacks and mulattoes in Peru, who had anxiously been awaiting the constitutional decision on their citizenship rights. On 10 March 1812 – just nine days before the promulgation of the Cádiz Constitution – there appeared in the newspaper *El Peruano* an article signed by "a descendant from Africa" who was still expecting full citizenship rights to be granted to all ethnic groups within the empire. Claiming that his parents had arrived in Peru from the Kingdom of Congo, the author confessed that he had experienced emotions that he had never felt before while reading the transcripts of the constitutional debates, especially the speeches made by some delegates in defence of the political rights of African descendants.[11] Their words had raised his expectations that the *castas* were about to be considered part of the Spanish nation in a way that had never been possible. Excited and full of anticipation, he asked the many blacks, mulattos, *zambos*, and *chinos* of Lima to prepare themselves to receive "with humble gratitude the sovereign decrees that come from Spain for our relief and happiness," but also to behave prudently until it became clear "what the courts have granted and, if necessary, we will petition with due respect that which proves useful and beneficial to us and to the state" (*El Peruano*, 10 March 1812; Morán Ramos 2008, 174). But it was not meant to be. The promulgation of the constitution in Lima in October of 1812 and the provisions established by Article 22 deeply disappointed the free blacks and mulattoes of Lima. Taking advantage of the 1811 decree that had established freedom of the press in the Spanish empire, some of them decided to appeal to public opinion by printing leaflets severely criticizing this constitutional provision (McEvoy Carreras 2002, 837).[12]

One of the most significant texts to emerge in this context was a work entitled *Reflexiones políticas y morales de un descendiente de África a su nación en que manifiesta sus amorosas quejas a los americanos sus hermanos*. Printed by Bernardino Ruiz at the Imprenta de los Huérfanos, *Reflexiones políticas y morales* was a short text that must have originally been written in verse, given the large number of internal rhymes; the verse was preceded by a brief introduction written in Latin.[13] It was printed anonymously by an individual who identified himself as a *pardo*. The only Peruvian *pardo* known to have a good command of Latin and to have previously published historical and political poetry – as we have seen – José Pastor de Larrinaga. Moreover, the opinions defended in *Reflexiones políticas y morales* on the issues of race, slavery, and the political rights of Afro-descendants were strikingly similar in tone and content to those already expressed by Larrinaga in his *Apología de los cirujanos del Perú*.

The author of *Reflexiones políticas y morales* began his discourse by reclaiming the rights of blacks and mulattoes to speak and be heard in colonial society: "Everyone talks, everyone writes, everyone asks for their rights. Only my people are silent, but there is a time to speak and a time to be quiet. Now is no longer the time to hold one's tongue, but the time to demand, as other nations do, the restoration of our rights. If we do not demand them, who will? And, if we do not speak, who will speak for us?" (*Reflexiones*, 2). He denounced the fact that Afro-descendants had been deprived of their citizenship rights and had not even been consulted on the issue. Moreover, as he reminded his Spanish American "brothers," none of those who represented Peru at the Cortes de Cádiz "were elected by us, since we lacked a voice in the voting process" (*Reflexiones*, 7 fn; see also Paniagua Corazao 2003, 80–109). To deny Afro-descendants the right to vote was a moral injustice, based on the mistaken idea that Nature had endowed other races with intellectual gifts and abilities that "are not found with equal perfection in us" (*Reflexiones*, 2). As for the conditions under which the Cortes de Cádiz would permit citizenship to be granted to blacks and mulattoes, he labelled them "metaphysical impossibilities," given the marginalized socio-economic status of that segment of the population. In a radical libertarian tone, highly reminiscent of Larrinaga's *Apología de los cirujanos del Perú*, the author argued that all men were born equal and free, according to both religion and natural law. Consequently, they should benefit from the same civil rights. He pointed out the cruel irony implied in enslaving their ancestors under the pretense of "civilizing" them – or, as the author sarcastically put it, "of making them as happy as other citizens" – only to deny them afterwards the same constitutional rights that those other citizens enjoyed in terms of political participation and access to employment and education (*Reflexiones*, 6). He concluded by remarking that despite directing his discourse to his compatriots, he no longer harboured any hope that his arguments might somehow move his white peers to join the cause of the *castas*. On the contrary, blacks and mulattoes would be more likely to find sympathy for their plight among the Indians than among those "who have nourished themselves with our milk and still subsist on our blood" (*Reflexiones*, 9).

A second, longer, and more sophisticated text also appeared in 1812, entitled *Colección de los discursos que pronunciaron los señores diputados de América contra el artículo 22 del proyecto de Constitución: Ilustrado con algunas notas interesantes por los españoles pardos de esta capital*. Also published by Bernardino Ruiz at the Imprenta de los Huérfanos, the book was an extensively annotated transcription of the speeches given by American representatives at the Cortes de Cádiz against the *de facto* exclusion of blacks and mulattoes from Spanish citizenship. As signalled in the title, it was edited by a group of *españoles pardos* who resided in Lima. Who exactly those *españoles pardos* were is not mentioned in the book, but given the substantial space they devoted to the achievements of Lima's *pardo* surgeons and physicians, it is likely that the authors came from this professional group. It is highly probable that doctors such as Valdés and others whose names and works figured prominently in the book were aware of its contents and may have contributed to it, given their support for the Cádiz liberal regime. Finally, it is also possible that both texts, *Reflexiones políticas y morales* and the *Colección de los dicursos*, were connected at least in their origin, since there is a clear overlap in the arguments used by the authors.

Like the author of *Reflexiones políticas y morales*, the editors of the *Colección de los discursos* attributed the exclusion of blacks and mulattoes from Spanish citizenship to the bigoted views that many individuals in Spain and America still held on the issue of race, and they wondered what catalyzed such shameful and humiliating prejudice: "Maybe their African origins?... Maybe their colour?... Maybe their alledged immorality and ignorance, as some representatives claim? Or is it by chance the slavery suffered by their ancestors that degrades them so much? And, if so, what blame can be placed on their grandparents for having been deprived of their freedom by rapacious and inhuman hands?" (*Colección*, iii). Adding insult to injury, the Cádiz Constitution included provisions that facilitated the process of granting Spanish citizenship to foreign nationals – even in the case of those who came from countries that were traditionally enemies of Spain. The editors considered this such a flagrant injustice that they did not hesitate to affirm that "if a flame of the most pure, generous, and noble patriotism did not burn in our chests, we might well prefer to have been born French rather than Spanish" (ibid., ii).

To prefer to have been born French rather than Spanish was quite a statement, given that Spain was at war with France. Nevertheless, the ideas expressed in *Colección de los discursos* were in general less confrontational than those defended in *Reflexiones políticas y morales*, and the editors preferred to reaffirm their allegiance rather than seeing it questioned. In this regard, they presented themselves as dependable subjects who had served the king on many occasions, guarding the coast of the viceroyalty against foreign pirates, putting down indigenous rebellions, and relieving the strain on the Royal Treasury (*Diario de las discusiones y actas de las Cortes* VIII, 4 de septiembre–7 de septiembre de 1811, 143–225; *Colección de los discursos* 1812, 40n16). They were outraged at the mere suggestion that they might join the rebels following the example of Caracas and Buenos Aires if they were not granted full citizenship rights, "because we are more worthy of esteem on account of our loyalty and virtue than we would be as citizens with neither of those qualities" (*Colección*, 65n20). To those who still expressed doubts, they replied with indignation: "Our loyalty is unwavering; and, as such, denying us the right to citizenship will never produce any other effects than those that are already known. Namely, to ask humbly for what in all fairness belongs to us and to redouble our efforts to prove our virtue, honesty, and patriotism" (*Colección*, 8n3). They wholeheartedly supported the proposal of representative Arizpe who asked the Cortes not only to grant Spanish citizenship to Afrodescendants but also to scrap the caste system completely and erase from "our laws and even from our public papers those hateful names: gachupin, creole, indian, mulato, etc." (*Colección*, 30). They believed the proposal to be "most just and necessary," since without "the proscription of those hateful names, we will never achieve the equality and unity that we so desire" (30n13).

In order to strenghten their case, the editors of the *Colección de los discursos* chose to underline the many contributions they had made to the progress of the colonies. Medicine ranked high among them. In his speech at the Cortes, the Peruvian delegate of indigenous descent, Dionisio Inca Yupanqui, had praised the work done by the black surgeons and doctors of Lima (*Colección*, 92–104).[14] The editors seized this opportunity to comment on the participation of blacks and mulattoes in public health, crediting them for the advancements made in surgery and medicine in the viceroyalty, "which probably would not have happened if whites alone had been practising those disciplines" (*Colección*, 90n24). Ever since the time of the mulatto surgeon Pedro de Utrilla, they argued, Afro-Peruvian surgeons, such as Larrinaga, Salas, Castell, Cáceres, Ávila, and Montero, had performed complex surgical interventions without having to enlist the help of their European counterparts. They had also assisted midwives in difficult pregnancies and childbirths that white doctors often refused to take care of (*Colección*, 98). Afro-Peruvians had become successful doctors as well as surgeons, and despite the limitations established by the Royal Decree of 1752, they insisted that there had always been "among the professors of the Faculty of Medicine at San Marcos a few who were descended from Africa" (*Colección*, 90n24]). Most of the editors' praise went to José Manuel Dávalos and José Manuel Valdés, to whom they devoted extensive biographical notes, but they also mentioned the contribution made by two lesser-known figures, José María Dávila and José Puente.

As news of the promulgation of the constitution finally reached Peru, the editors of the *Colección* bitterly complained that the final wording of Article 22 made it very difficult for these accomplished physicians – and almost impossible for any other person of African ancestry – to obtain full rights as citizens of the empire (*Colección*, 115). Despite this, not all news arriving from Cádiz in 1812 boded poorly for Afro-descendants. Shortly after the promulgation of the constitution, it became known in Lima that the Cortes had signed a decree that effectively dismantled the existing *casta* legislation and granted blacks and mulattoes a number of rights, including the right to attend the schools and universities of their choice, to be ordained as priests –provided they satisfied the requirements established by canon law – and to practise any profession for which they were sufficiently qualified (*Diario de las discusiones y actas de las Cortes* XI, 26 de enero de 1812, 392; *Colección de los discursos* 1812, 117). By issuing this decree, the Cortes addressed – albeit outside the constitutional text – some of the main complaints of the American delegates and gave the *castas* a chance to obtain Spanish citizenship through the process outlined in Article 22. Of course, it was still possible to exploit legal ambiguities and other loopholes to undermine the attempts of people of African ancestry to advance professionally or politically in colonial society; but the decree was seen as an almost revolutionary change from previous legislation. It must have been made public in Lima just as the *Colección* was about to hit the press, since it prompted the editors to include a hurried but joyful final note: "As soon as we learned of this unexpected gift, our hearts were filled with the most tender gratitude to the Almighty ... and we rejoiced upon seeing the doors of enlightment and honour finally opened" (*Colección*, 118). As a way of showing their loyalty to the metropolis and their appreciation for the new legislation, the editors resolved to offer a mass in the name of the *españoles pardos* of Lima to ask God "for the triumph of the royal armies throughout the Spanish monarchy," and they swore "to spill their blood in defence of their country in case of need" (119).

The educated *pardos* and *mulatos* who qualified for Spanish citizenship did not have to wait long for a chance to exercise what they saw as their legitimate political rights. The opportunity arose with a mandate issued by the Cortes to renew all city councils through a popular vote, in line with statutes that had been established by the new constitution. In Lima, the voters divided into two groups: those in favour of the candidates proposed by Viceroy Abascal, who supported the traditional absolutist status quo, and those more inclined towards political and constitutional reform, who grouped around the leadership of the Audiencia's prosecutor Miguel Eyzaguirre (Paniagua Corazao 2003, 183–8). As was expected, one of the problems was to establish who could vote and who could not, according to the provisions of the Cádiz Constitution (Peralta Ruiz 2008, 70). The *Censo general de la población de Lima hecho a fines del año de 1812* confusingly divided the population of the city into "citizens with voting rights" (5,243), "citizens without voting rights" (6,670), "female citizens" (11,460), "male Spaniards" (7,871), "female Spaniards" (11,239), "clergy" (959), "nuns" (473), "male slaves" (6,400), "female slaves" (5,863), and "foreigners" (106) (AGI, Lima 747; in Anna 1975, 236).[15] Most blacks and mulattoes must have been considered either "slaves" or "citizens without voting rights"; as such, they were not authorized to participate in the election. Despite this, complaints were made throughout the process, claiming that many Afro-descendants as well as under-age individuals had been allowed to vote (Peralta Ruiz 2008, 78). Tensions grew as it became clear that those headed by Eyzaguirre had won the election, and Abascal accused him of meddling with the parish voting process for his own benefit (Anna 1979, 59; Hamnet 2000, 12).

For their part, blacks and mulattoes seem to have greeted the outcome of the election with enthusiasm. Among those who expressed satisfaction was José Manuel Valdés. On 25 February 1813 he published an ode in the newspaper *El verdadero peruano* extolling the importance of the right to vote.[16] He called the election a "memorable day / for me unforgettable," when the people of Lima could finally consider themselves free, having happily avoided – unlike other parts of the Americas – the ravages of war, that "frightening deluge / in which kingdoms and cities are wrecked" (Valdés 1813, 224–5). The only thing detracting from the complete happiness of Lima's residents was the granting of equal rights to all. In a clear allusion to the constitutional debates on citizenship, Valdés asked rhetorically why the motherland still denied "such a privilege to those who for two hundred years have given constant proof of their unfailing love" (225). But dismissing legal inequality as merely temporary, with its amelioration inevitable, Valdés predicted a future of political stability and economic prosperity for the viceroyalty and for the Spanish empire as a whole. Miners would extract the hidden metals that mountains hide "in their horrid interiors," commerce "would flourish," and science and art would enlighten regions "that rivers of blood have now turned dark" (227–8). His poem was accompanied by a note from the editors of *El verdadero peruano* supporting the ideas he expressed and advocating that the *pardos* of the city be "decorated with the noble insignia of Spanish citizens" for the "many services that their talent and courage have rendered to the fatherland" (228).

Not everybody shared the optimism of *El verdadero peruano* or interpreted the political participation of the *castas* as a positive development. Months after the election of the new city council, the newspaper *El Investigador del Perú* still questioned the political role the *castas* had played in the election and criticized the sympathy that the city council showed towards them. It decried that ever since then, Lima had become infested with thieves, many of whom were "ferocious Africans" (*El Investigador*, 30–31 October 1813, 237–44; ibid., 19 July 1814, 3–4). A letter in the newspaper in July 1814 asked how it was possible that free blacks had become the true legislators of the capital of Peru and complained that there was no "position these people did not attempt to fill without anyone daring to put them in their proper place as non-citizens" (*El Investigador*, 25 July 1814, 4). In August the newspaper denounced the fact that many *pardos* had been elected to the city council of Samborondón, near Guayaquil, in spite of their race and their reputation as "inept, barbaric, and despicable men" (*El Investigador*, 26 August 1814, 4).

Unfortunately for Valdés and for those who saw in the newly elected city council the dawn of a new day, the situation in Lima did not please Viceroy Abascal. He did not declare the results of the election void – as Viceroy Benegas had done in New Spain – but with the support of the Audiencia de Lima and the Diputación provincial he did succeed in excluding Eyzaguirre from politics by applying a constitutional article that prohibited court prosecutors from holding constitutional positions. Without their leader, and lacking the support of the institutions controlled by the viceroy, the city council could hardly fulfill the obligations conferred on it by the Constitution of 1812, and it dissolved halfway through 1814 (Peralta Ruiz 2008, 78). Abascal again called for elections to the Cabildo and again *El Investigador del Perú* denounced the illegitimate participation of people of African descent in the electoral process. Reminding the viceroy that the people of Lima were not satisfied with what had occurred in those elections, the newspaper asked to repeat the election "not among mulatos but Spanish citizens, as it should be, since we would otherwise be entering a labyrinth in which even the blacks could vote" (*El Investigador*, 15 November 1814, 1). There was no time for a new vote. The return of Ferdinand VII to the throne of Spain meant the end of the Constitution of 1812 and the reimposition of absolute monarchy both in the metropolis and in Peru.

Royalists, Patriots, and Doctors

On 6 September 1814, while Ferdinand VII destroyed the last remains of the Cádiz liberal regime, Larrinaga wrote an enthusiastic letter to the Cabildo proposing the erection of a bronze statue of the king on horseback to honour his return (Larrinaga 1814). Larrinaga had entertained this "sublime and happy idea" as early as 1812 in his *Cartas históricas a un amigo*. He suggested that the statue be placed in a new city square "with an iron fence completely surrounded by metal plates engraved with the poems and hieroglyphs about the loss and restoration of Spain that [his] limited talent had been able to devise" (Larrinaga 1812, 161–2). In front of the statue, Larrinaga proposed to build a new church under the invocation of St Ferdinand, where "our Sociedad patriótica del Monte pío de los cirujanos will celebrate each year a solemn office to thank God for the glorious triumphs of our armies, followed the next day by a requiem mass in honour of those who had fallen defending the fatherland" (ibid., 162).

Larrinaga made no secret of his political inclinations. He had held Ferdinand VII "in my heart," he declared, since the day the king was born. He revealed that he had written his poems on the history of the Incas and the Spanish rulers of Peru that appeared in the *Mercurio peruano* in 1792 in order to educate the young prince in the art of ruling an empire (Larrinaga 1812, 161). Upon learning of France's invasion of Spain, he had "electrified" his contemporaries with some *décimas* [a ten-line, octosyllabic poem] denouncing the illegitimacy of Ferdinand VII's abdication and calling on his fellow compatriots to rise in arms against Napoleon, whom he referred to as a "man-eating wolf" (quoted in Rabí Chara 2006b, 227; Larrinaga 1812, 161). Larrinaga even reinterpreted Asunción's extraordinary birth of a pigeon from a political and eschatological point of view, claiming that the monster born in Lima in the form of a bird "with no head, no neck, no wings, and no legs" foretold "the ruin of Spain itself, with Charles IV lacking a head to think, without wings to do what is right, without legs to act on his own, and with no other neck than that of the shameful Godoy, who sacrificed all to his ambition, his glory, his greed, and his lasciviousness" (Larrinaga 1812, 152–3).[17]

Larrinaga's staunch support of King Ferdinand VII and absolute rule seems to contradict his position on slavery and the rights of Afrodescendants, but this is not necessarily so. He saw Viceroy Abascal and the *criollo* elite, personified by the protomédicos Juan José de Aguirre and Hipólito Unanue, as his main enemies. Like other colonial subjects who found themselves at odds with the viceregal authorities, he presented himself as a loyal servant of the king in the hope of obtaining justice for the wrongdoings of his officials. In all fairness to Larrinaga, it must be said that most people in Lima shared – or at least pretended to share – his joy over the restoration of the monarchy. How many truly felt about the dissolution of the Cortes and the abrogation of the Cádiz Constitution is more difficult to discern. The return of absolutism in Peru resulted in an increase in the persecution of those with revolutionary and even reformist ideas. All the liberal newspapers that had appeared since 1811 were shut down, and the permission to print became tightly controlled once again (Martínez Riaza 1982, 133–4).

In the case of Unanue, the Absolutist Restoration caught him by surprise on his way to Spain after having been elected to the Cortes as a representative of Arequipa. Finding himself without a political mandate, he chose to concentrate his efforts on securing the final authorization for the Real Colegio de medicina y cirugía de San Fernando. After achieving this goal, he went back to Peru, arriving in Lima on 12 August 1816. Once there, he withdrew from active political life and resumed his medical and academic responsibilities. Dávalos and Valdés followed Unanue's example and, at least in public, accepted the return to absolute rule. During the celebrations that took place in Lima on 30 May 1814, Dávalos delivered a clearly pro-monarchical speech, in which he described society as "an inert and blind mass" that needed the guidance of the sovereign in order to receive "the direction most convenient to its own utility" (Dávalos 1815, 2). He assured colonial authorities that future generations of students at San Marcos would "learn to love our King and to reject the chimeras of freedom and independence spread by the rebels, in the knowledge that our august Monarch is naturally destined in the New World to rule over the great empire that extends from the Strait of Magellan to the Missisipi River" (ibid., 3–4). As for Valdés, his position and prestige in the medical world of absolutist Lima grew even further. By 1814, he was surgical examiner in the Tribunal del Protomedicato and chair of Clinical Medicine at the University of San Marcos. He was employed as a physician at the hospitals of San Pedro and San Juan de Dios; at the Royal Congregation of San Felipe Neri's Oratory; and at the convent and monastery of Santa Catalina and San Francisco. According to Lavalle, his clientele came "from the most powerful and aristocratic homes, from the highest public employees, and from the most distinguished members of the clergy," – that is, from those sectors of the Peruvian elite that most strongly supported Ferdinand VII's restoration (Lavalle n.d., 15).[18]

Despite their professional successes and the lip service paid to colonial authorities, the political ideas of Valdés and Dávalos' – like those of many other doctors – probably became more radical between the return of Ferdinand VII to the Spanish throne in 1814 and the triumphant entry of General José de San Martín into Lima in 1821. Many historians have viewed the Colegio de medicina y cirugía de San Fernando, where both Dávalos and Valdés taught, as a hotbed of revolutionary thought in the years preceding Peruvian independence (Pamo Reina 2009, 62). Miguel Tafur provided further evidence of the revolutionary leanings of the college when he read a discourse in 1822 suggesting that the institution created by Unanue had secretly harboured Peruvian patriots persecuted by the Spaniards (ibid.). The radicalization of some segments of the Peruvian intellectual and economic elite was no doubt influenced by the fiscal collapse of the viceroyalty and the weakening of commerce in the Pacific. By the time Viceroy Abascal returned to Spain in 1816, the viceroyalty had an accumulated debt of eleven million pesos (Hamnet 2000, 15).

The situation deteriorated further in the years following Abascal's departure. In 1818 an epidemic ravaged the city, causing many of its residents to fall ill with fever, diarrhea, and vomiting. As one of the city's leading doctors, Valdés was among those consulted about the possible causes of the sickness. He did his best to reinforce the official explanation, which blamed the fevers and the increased mortality rate on an especially hot and humid summer. He did not, however, hesitate to point to the widespread poverty and the bad quality of meat and bread as elements that considerably contributed to the effect of the fever. He also called on the viceregal authorities to initiate a campaign to counter the abysmal hygienic conditions of the city and to supervise the capital's food distribution chain more closely (Valdés 1840, 140).[19] Despite this, the situation became worse as time went by. Valdés later recalled the terrible days that preceded the fall of Lima to San Martín's troops. He did so in a text that is significant not only as an illustration of Valdés's process of portraying himself as a doctor and a patriot, but as one of the few descriptions of the Peruvian War of Independence written by a person of African descent:

> Consider our situation before the happy day when the king's army left this city. Such contrasts in ten months under siege! What changing feelings on both sides! How many scenes of pain brought about by a war whose success always seemed so doubtful! The tyrants and their proxies were moved by hatred and rage

and the patriots by fear and mistrust. The former spied on the victims they sought to sacrifice to their fury; the latter found it necessary to avoid being caught and to bring the business they had started to a conclusion. There were those who cried for their parents, for their children, or for their wives, either dead or held prisoner during the campaign or at risk of perishing in the gallows on account of their opinions; others voluntarily exiled themselves; while still others passed away in the company of their dear and tender children destined to die in poverty. Fear overtook the population on account of the spread of a rumour indicating that the liberating army would loot the city if allowed to get it; and so both patriot and royalist families feared equally becoming victims of the ferocious militiamen enforcing the siege. The exit of the royal army filled the hearts of those who loved their country with joy, but it was very bitter for many people who were bound to the king's troops by blood, friendship, and gratitude. Some desired their return and triumph, while others were frighten of it. Hearts fluctuated between fear and hope until that memorable day, the seventh of September, when the people of Lima, protected by the liberating army and animated by heroic enthusiasm, made the Spanish troops tremble to the point of convincing them that their return was entirely impossible. That sadness and fear facilitate the development of grave and malignant illnesses – sometimes leading even to death – is such a well-known fact that it would be futile to prove it. Even after achieving our independence, the sadness of the preceding years continued to devastate many poor and unsettled families. My dear friend Doctor Paredes and I had the occasion to witness the unfortunate death of a young woman who became sick with a spasmodic form of putrid fever caused by the imprisonment of her husband. By the time he was freed, she was already delirious. We took the precaution of letting her know about his freedom before allowing him to see her. He entered the room and spoke to her with a tenderness inspired by the love in his tortured heart. She opened her eyes, answered him, and seemed to become happier at his sight; but immediately afterwards she fell into a rapture that left her body bathed in an icy sweat, passing away in the arms of the dear object of her affections. (Valdés 1827, 30)

In spite of the hardships of the siege, many of the city's inhabitants greeted San Martín's triumphant entry into Lima with enthusiasm. On 15 July 1821, a formal declaration of independence was drafted by the city council proclaiming that "the general will is decided in favor of the Independence of Peru from Spanish domination, and that of whatever other foreign power" (Odriozola 1877, 38; translation by Anna 1975, 221). It was signed by many of the city's most distinguished citizens, including Hipólito Unanue, Miguel Tafur, José Pezet, and José Manuel Dávalos (Pamo Reina 2009, 63; Odriozola 1877, 39).[20] Making use of revolutionary rhetoric that he had not employed in public until then, Valdés wrote an ode to the liberator of Peru in which he praised all those who had fought and fallen for the cause of liberty, calling them "valiant patriots who purged / the earth of tyrants and who killed / the ferocious beasts" (Valdés 1871, 764). He depicted General José de San Martín as a providential figure charged by Heaven with the mission of liberating Peru, who had rightly assumed leadership "until the clear day dawns / when a benevolent government is established / that determines the country's destiny" (ibid., 766).

San Martín responded to these and other enthusiastic demonstrations of support by bestowing numerous honours on Lima's doctors. The Colegio de medicina y cirugía de San Fernando, where many of them taught, was renamed Colegio de la Independencia, a designation that lasted until 1856, when Peruvian higher education was reorganized and the institution changed its name to the Facultad de medecina de San Marcos (Delgado Matallana & Rabí Chara 2006, 83). Hipólito Unanue was decorated with the highest degree of the newly created Order of the Sun (*grado de fundador*), a distinction created to honour those who had distinguished themselves for their contributions to the cause of independence. José Pezet and José Manuel Valdés were also awarded the Order of the Sun, but in a lower category (*grado de asociado*).[21] Doctors also benefited both socially and professionally from San Martín's government: Unanue became finance minister, and Valdés was designated Médico de Cámara del gobierno (Lavalle n.d., 16). Before leaving to meet Simón Bolívar at Guayaquil in July of 1822, the Argentine general also made Unanue vice-president and named Valdés a permanent member of the short-lived Sociedad patriótica, a learned society whose mission was the social, economic, and political advancement of Peru (Lavalle n.d., 16).[22]

San Martín's resignation as "Protector of Peru" on 20 September 1822 was followed by a period of grave institutional instability, characterized by the constant fear of a Spanish counteroffensive. Called on by the Peruvian Congress to take care of military operations in the country, Bolívar left Guayaquil and was enthusiastically received in Lima on 1 September 1823. One of his first actions in Peru was to deal with the deposed president, José de la Riva Agüero,[23] who had decreed from Trujillo the dissolution of Congress and was secretly negotiating a truce with the Spaniards. With this enemy out of the way, the Venezuelan general concentrated on the task of expelling the Spanish troops commanded by Viceroy José de la Serna. A series of political and military setbacks, including the revolt of the garrison of Callao and the occupation of Lima by royalist troops, forced the Peruvian Congress to suspend the constitution and appoint Bolívar as dictator of Peru on 10 February 1824. Armed with these new powers, Bolívar was able to reorganize his army and inflict a serious defeat on the Spanish forces at the battle of Junín on 6 August 1824. A few months later, on 9 December, Antonio José de Sucre, Bolívar's lieutenant, destroyed the remaining Spanish army at the battle of Ayacucho, thereby securing the independence of Peru. Just two days before that fateful battle, Bolívar had entered Lima – which had been abandoned by the royalist forces after receiving news of the defeat at Junín – amid the loudest acclamations of its inhabitants.

Among those who celebrated Bolívar's return was José Manuel Valdés, who dedicated a poem to him entitled "Lima libre y pacífica" (Valdés 1825, n.p.). As he had previously done with San Martín, Valdés presented the *Libertador* as an auspicious and heroic figure. He was chosen by God to defend the Christian religion and "destroy the old irons" that once again had chained the capital of Peru to the Spanish king (ibid., 4). Valdés depicted him as a "tempest of formidable rays" who defended the country against its internal and external enemies and put an end to "the horrors produced by hatred, impiety, hunger, and war, which had made the world a miserable place" (1). Bolívar's final triumph, wrote Valdés, was the best guarantee for the future establishment of a "fatherly and fair government" that would promote religion, the sciences, and the arts (8–9). But the deteriorating political situation in Colombia made Bolívar's presence in Peru untenable, and he left the country in 1826, though not without first establishing a short-lived *constitución vitalicia* (life constitution) for both Peru and the newly created country of Bolivia.

After Bolívar's departure, Valdés became more and more actively involved in the uncertain field of Peruvian politics. He was even elected *diputado suplente* by the province of Lima in 1828 (Lavalle n.d., 18). But it did not take long for him to convince himself that his future was not in Congress. He returned to the university, where he had been named chair of Vísperas de medicina, and rose to further prominence at the Protomedicato, where he served under the protomédico Miguel Tafur. By then, his colleagues José Pastor de Larrinaga and José Manuel Dávalos had died. Larrinaga had passed away at some point between 1821 and 1823. Lima's medical establishment does not seem to have noticed his absence, for no funeral eulogy was publicly recorded and even his death certificate is lost (Rabi Chara 2006, 28). As for José Manuel Dávalos, he must have died shortly after the proclamation of independence: he dictated his final will and testament to the public notary, Juan Pio de Espinosa, on 22 October 1821 (Dávalos 1821; Lastres 1955, 168; Vargas Ugarte 1943, 325–42). Thus, of the three most distinguished mulatto physicians of the period, only José Manuel Valdés remained by the end of the 1820s. In the following decade, he would crown his already extraordinary career by becoming Protomédico general de la República, the highest honour ever bestowed upon an Afro-descendant in early republican Peru.

CHAPTER 4

A Black Protomédico in Republican Peru

Following Peru's independence from Spain in 1821, the Real Tribunal del Protomedicato was transformed into the Protomedicato general de la República. Unanue's active role in the emancipation process and in the governments that emerged after independence opened the directorship of the new office to Miguel Tafur, who filled in as substitute protomédico until 1826, when he officially took the position on a permanent basis (Bustios Romani 2004, 302).[1] Nevertheless, Unanue's influence continued to be felt on various public health issues at least until 1827, when he decided to retire from public life and move to his *hacienda* in Cañete. Up to that point, Unanue had spearheaded legislation regulating the protection of children (1821), the functioning of military hospitals (1825), the work of slaves (1825), the Juntas de sanidad (1826), the Dirección general de beneficencia (1826), the maternity house (1826), and the reports on the country's demographics (1826) and vaccination campaigns (1826) (Bustios Romani 2004, 252). Given Unanue's legislative activity, Tafur considered that his main obligation as protomédico was to ensure that the many institutional transformations taking place in the new republic did not affect the main roles of his office. Consequently, the Protomedicato continued to make certain that no one could engage in the practice of medicine without the proper degrees and licences, as in colonial times. It also tried to make certain that doctors and apothecaries practised their profession according to what the old tribunal had considered best practice. Valdés became Tafur's right hand and then protomédico himself in 1835, less than two years after the death of his colleague.

Tafur's and Valdés's determination was soon tested by the Franciscan priest Juan Joseph Matraya y Ricci's introduction in Peru of the "curative method" promoted by the French surgeon Louis Leroy, along with Leroy's "panchymagogue," a supposedly miraculous drug able to cure almost any illness. What was soon known as "the Matraya affair" convinced them that it was more necessary than ever to strengthen the authority of their office in the treacherous scientific and political environment of early republican Peru. They sought to do so both legally – by countering the legislation that sought to weaken the powers of the Protomedicato – and intellectually – by making their office the champion of "Peruvian medicine." In this regard, and following Unanue's vision, their aim was to establish a body of medical knowledge best suited to the kinds of illness most prevalent in Peru and specifically tailored to the climate and other physical characteristics of the country. In their dependence on the work of Hipólito Unanue, Tafur and Valdés's scientific views were not particularly innovative. But even if their ideas were far from original, the sociopolitical context in which they were expressed was very different from that of 1805, when Unanue had published his *Observaciones sobre el clima de Lima*. Doctors such as Tafur and Valdés saw themselves as the proud representatives of scientific medicine in the new nation, particularly after Unanue's retirement. They harboured the ambition of elevating Peruvian medicine to the heights of its European counterparts and sought to impose their authority and conception of medicine on all practitioners, both national and foreign. These projects were challenged, first by Matraya y Ricci and his defence of Leroy's panchimagoge; then by a folk healer named Dorotea Salguero and her surprisingly fierce liberal allies; and finally by an English doctor, Archibald Smith, and those – both inside and outside the Peruvian medical establishment – who called for the end of the Protomedicato. Valdés's tenure as protomédico was therefore marked by great controversy. While many doctors saw Valdés's actions against folk healers and foreign physicians as protecting not only an endogenous medical tradition but also their economic interests, a growing number rejected the complete supervision of their medical practice that Valdés sought to impose as a trade-off for his protectionism.

Tafur, Valdés, and the Panchymagogue

The Matraya affair began in 1825 when news reached the Protomédicato general de la República that a Franciscan priest named Juan Joseph Matraya y Ricci claimed to have the key to cure all sorts of maladies. As noted above, the priest's revolutionary method was based on the theories of the French surgeon Louis Leroy, whose work *La médecine naturelle et curative, ou La purgation dirigée contre la cause des maladies* [Curative medicine, or, purgation, directed against the cause of diseases] had appeared in Paris in 1817. Leroy's book soon became very popular in both Europe and America. A Spanish translation with the title *La medicina curativa, ó, La purgacion dirigida contra la causa de las enfermedades* appeared in 1820 in Valencia (Imprenta de Ildefonso Mompie), in 1824 in Buenos Aires (Imprenta de Hallet), in 1833 in Mexico (Imprenta de Galván), and it was still in print in Lima as late as 1852 (Imprenta de los Sres. Calleja, Ojea y Compañía). Leroy's medical ideas were in turn based on the experiences of his father-in-law, a health officer named Jean Pelgas (1732–1804). Their system, aptly named purgative and vomi-purgative, rested on a medical conception similar to that of popular humoralism – namely, that the body contained in itself the germ of its own destruction, which needed to be expunged if it was to remain healthy (Ramsey 1992, 118–19). In order to achieve this goal, they administered two remedies of their own invention (manufactured in Paris by the pharmacist Cottin, who happened to be Leroy's son-in-law). These preparations "were the best known and probably the most destructive pharmaceutical specialties of early-nineteenth-century France … The purgative, available in several 'degrees' (strengths), was described as a tincture of scammony, turpeth root, and jalap root; the vomi-purgative contained senna extract, tartar emetic, and white wine" (Ramsey 1994, 42).

Others had tried to introduce universal remedies to Lima and other parts of the Spanish empire before (Lanning 1985, 362–6), but the case of Leroy's universal medicine, or *panquimagogo* as it was called in Spanish, was different on several counts. First, "such aggressive therapies won wide acceptance because they demonstrably worked in the sense of producing visible results (purges really purged), and because their actions made sense within a shared system of explanation" (Ramsey 1994, 42). Moreover, they came imbued with the prestige of European and particularly French science. It was supported by the work of doctors and surgeons who claimed to have found a new scientific paradigm far superior to all the competing medical theories of the time. In this regard, Leroy "always distinguished between his own curative medicine and official medicine, which was merely palliative" (ibid., 43). Finally, the very diffusion of Leroy's book and many others that were based on it gave his system an aura of learning, respectability, and acceptance that distinguished him from the remedies sold in the streets by folk healers and quacks. His book was sold at a very low price by mail order, and this, too, helped Leroy to gain a wide audience. (ibid., 42).

Leroy's champion in Peru was no ignoramus himself. Juan Joseph Matraya y Ricci was an influential member of the church, well versed in different disciplines, but especially in law. He was the author of the compilation of laws *Catálogo cronológico de pragmáticas, céduas, decretos, órdenes y resoluciones reales* (1819) as well as of the treatise *El moralista filalethico americano, o El confesor imparcial instruido en las obligaciones de su Ministerio según los preceptos de la más sólida theología moral* (1819). According to his testimony, he had obtained a copy of Leroy's book in early 1825 and had begun to distribute the panchymagoge immediately after witnessing its beneficial effects. The Protomedicato immediately forbade apothecaries to prepare the remedy ordered by the priest and asked him to cease his medical activities. Far from backing down, Matraya began to manufacture the remedy himself and even wrote a summary of Leroy's work in which he provided practical advice for its administration (Matraya y Ricci 1825a, 1). On 21 October 1825, Tafur finally asked the provincial head of the Franciscan Order to forbid Father Matraya from practising medicine and prescribing the panchymagoge, since it was "an empirical remedy extraordinarily harmful in the hands of an unskilled person," whose untimely and misguided administration had considerably aggravated the condition of many patients (ibid.). Tafur considered it entirely unfitting of the "decency and decorum owed to his ministry" that "a priest and man of God should act as a folk healer" (ibid.).

Matraya's answer appeared in a public letter addressed to the Protomedicato entitled *Defensa de la medicina curativa y lícita administración de su único remedio nombrado panquimagogo por cualquiera instruido en su dirección práctica aunque sea clérigo o religioso* (1825). In this text, Matraya justified his actions on religious and scientific grounds. From the point of view of religion, he argued that there was no contradiction between his work as a priest and as a doctor. Christ himself had sent his disciples to preach the Kingdom of God and cure the sick, and as recently as 1748, Pope Benedict XIV had ordered missionaries to study and practise medicine, "since curing the body's illnesses was the most conducive means to win over the souls of men for Christ" (ibid.). As for the validity of Leroy's theories, he considered that the French doctor had demonstrated "scientifically and experimentally that there is no time, condition, or circumstance in the life of a man in which his remedies cannot and should not be administered" (ibid., 2). To emphasize the experimental validity of Leroy's medicines and to refute Tafur's accusations, Matraya himself provided at the end of his text a long list of names of patients in Lima who had recovered their health thanks to the universal curative properties of the panchymagoge.

In view of this public challenge, Tafur once again wrote to Matraya's superior, asking him to control the rebellious priest and warning him that unless Matraya ceased all his medical activities, the Protomedicato would enforce the laws concerning quacks and folk healers, which carried with them not only fines and possibly prison, but also expulsion from the city (Matraya 1825b, 1). Far from being intimidated, Matraya answered by publishing yet another, even more defiant text, entitled *Triunfo de la medicina curativa de Mr Leroy sobre la paliativa, dirigido al Sr. D. Miguel Tafur, Protomédico de Lima*. Matraya defended himself using a political argument that would resurface years later, one that illustrates the difficult legal and political context in which the office of the Protomedicato found itself during the first decades after emancipation. He reminded Tafur that independence had brought a new beginning, ending the times "when the doctor who obtained the viceroy's favour could govern the viceroyalty as he saw fit" (ibid., 2). As for Tafur's legal threats, he asked the Protomédico what exactly he thought he could do against him according to the law before. "Nothing; nothing; nothing," he declared (ibid.). Arguing again from a scientific and public health perspective, he accused those who formed the Protomédicato of having condemned Leroy's curative medicine "because it cures those whom paliative medicine kills or keeps perpetually sick" and were afraid of losing the revenue they obtained from their ineffective remedies (ibid.). That, and no other, was the reason the doctors of Lima had so far declined to disprove Leroy's scientific arguments. He vowed to continue with his practice and informed Tafur that he planned to sell the remedy in a store close to the city's main square.

As he had threatened, Tafur began legal proceedings aimed at preventing Father Matraya from selling and prescribing Leroy's panchymagoge. Seeking to avoid a trial, Matraya attempted to ingratiate himself with the protomédico, but to no avail. He published a final letter in 1826 in which he decried Tafur's failure to respond to his efforts at reconciliation and challenged him and his colleagues to divide a hospital in two sections so that, if "after a period of 40 days, you and your collagues cure more patients than me, I will accept as punishment to be exiled from this Republic ... But if, with the help of God, which I expect since I defend the cause of the people, I were to cure more of them than you, I would impose upon you out of my generosity only the punishment of perpetual silence" (Matraya 1826, 5). The challenge most probably never took place. Regardless, he left Peru in 1827, later to become an influential figure in the Vatican, where he advised Pope Gregory XVI on the missionary enterprise and the need to repopulate missions in the New World (Langer 2009, 66). The Matraya affair and the controversy surrounding Leroy's "curative method" helped those who had positions of responsibility at the Protomedicato to solidify their opinion that the body of medical knowledge patiently amassed in the decades preceding independence was under siege and that it was of the utmost importance to defend it from both internal and external enemies. Both Tafur and Valdés considered it more necessary than ever to continue the path opened by Hipólito Unanue and create a Peruvian medicine that could withstand the attack of folk healers and foreign doctors alike and reinforce the position of their office. This resulted in the publication in 1827 of Valdés's book *Memoria sobre las enfermedades epidémicas que se padecieron en Lima el año de 1821*.

Valdés's *Memoria* was first and foremost an epidemiological essay, but it also articulated remarkably well an understanding of medicine that was fully endorsed by those who were at the helm of the most important medical institutions in the country. For Valdés, the field found itself far removed from the advances experienced by other scientific disciplines and characterized by "systems that compete among themselves, convert many followers, and dominate the scientific world for short periods of time" (Valdés 1827, 4). Peruvian students were quick to adopt the latest theories from the faculties of medicine at Montpellier, Edinburgh, and Leiden, frequently forgetting that sickness differ from one region to another and that therefore "the remedies and their timing, doses, and form of administration" must also be different. Mankind would greatly benefit, Valdés argued, if doctors were to work harder at perfecting the practice of medicine in their own countries instead of simply copying what had been done in others (ibid.). He praised "the likes of Salinas, Avendaño, Bueno, Aguirre, Cano, Moreno, and all the other medical luminaries of Lima" for having done just that, with no other stimulus than their own sense of honour and responsibility. Valdés saw his book as a contribution that followed in the footsteps of these reformers and not as a radical departure from their tradition. As Bueno and Unanue had done before him, Valdés argued that despite obvious anatomical and physiological commonalities, medicine was above all a region-specific discipline and therefore geography and climate were key factors in the study of bodily illnesses.[2]

Tafur commended Valdés's essay as "an exemplary study in its field" and the first of what he hoped would become a large collection of studies aimed at training future generations of Peruvian physicians. He viewed Valdés's treatise as an integral part of his vision for a forthcoming course on Peruvian medicine and announced that no student was to be allowed to take the medical exams "without first presenting a copy of this *Memoria* and of the other texts that were to follow it" (Valdés 1827, iv). Valdés's text was also praised in the strongest possible terms by Nicolás de Pierola, director of the Colegio de la Independencia – as the former Colegio de medicina y cirugía de San Fernando founded by Unanue was now called. In a letter recommending its publication, Pierola said the work was proof that "the time of the complete regeneration of Peruvian medicine had finally arrived" and claimed that the book's "healthy doctrines" and the "exactitude of its observations and descriptions" would help to expand the fame of Peruvian medicine and the reputation of the government beyond the country's borders (Valdés 1827, ii). He consequently asked the government not only to finance it but to force the faculty of the Colegio de la Independencia to buy a copy to contribute to the printing costs (ibid.). José María de Pando, Peru's minister of interior, fully endorsed Pierola's and Tafur's commendations, though he asked them to persuade rather than force their colleagues to buy a copy of the book, and he ordered the Treasury to provide the funds necessary for its publication (ibid.).

Those at the Protomedicato who, like Tafur, believed that the departure of Juan Joseph Matraya and the publication of Valdés's *Memoria sobre las enfermedades epidémicas* heralded the beginning of an era of institutional and intellectual stability were soon to be disappointed. Less than a year later, the Protomedicato's attempt to control the activities of a humble *curandera* named Dorotea Salguero rapidly escalated into a heated public discussion on the right to choose, the role of that office in republican Peru, and the conception of medicine defended by those who, like Valdés, intellectually supported the protomédico's decisions.

Folk Medicine and Political Liberalism

The case against Dorotea Salguero began in 1828, when she was jailed at the request of the protomédico Miguel Tafur. Folk healers like her had been present in Lima since early colonial times. Unanue blamed their proliferation on the weakness of Peruvian medicine and considered them a plague that caused more harm to the population of Peru "than all of the illnesses that have afflicted us taken together" (Unanue 1793a, 101–2). Despite these harsh words, traditional medical practitioners remained very popular after independence, and many in Lima trusted their judgment over that of doctors when confronted with life-threatening illness. Tafur probably expected that his decision to prosecute Dorotea would raise some complaints from her patients, but – after having warned her twice to cease her activities – he was determined to make an example of her. He accused her of practising medicine and selling cures without authorization and without any regard for her patients' lives. He also made clear that these charges would swiftly be followed by more serious ones, including fraud and murder (*Defensa* 1831, 4).

Dorotea vehemently contested the accusations. She did not deny that she had performed procedures of the kind usually reserved for surgeons and doctors, but she claimed to have done so at the request of her patients and only after their own physicians had concluded that they were beyond any hope of recovery. With regard to her "cures," she argued that they were completely harmless herbal remedies and not *medica-mentos de botica* – medicines to be produced under the direct supervision of a trained pharmacist. Consequently, her remedies were not subject to the supervision of the Protomedicato, nor did she need its authorization to sell them (*Defensa* 1831, 4–5). To counter Dorotea's claims, Tafur provided three witnesses – a doctor and two surgeons – who upheld the Protomedicato's version of the events. Given the social and professional status of the witnesses, their word was readily – and illegally, according to Dorotea's lawyer – taken at face value by the court, which decided to keep the folk healer under arrest. Nevertheless, as it could not be proved that she had deceived or killed anybody, she was let out of jail a few days later on condition that she would not practise medicine again (6).

The court's threats do not seem to have scared Dorotea. Two years later, in August 1830, José Manuel Valdés and two other doctors informed Miguel Tafur that she was once again performing unauthorized cures. According to their testimony, Dorotea had asked one of their patients, a certain Manuela Vidal, to stop taking the medicines they had prescribed for the treatment of acute colic. In its place, Dorotea recommended an enema and prescribed the patient a "spirit" of her own invention, charging Manuela 20 reales for it. Outraged, Valdés and his colleagues demanded Dorotea's immediate prosecution in order to protect the life of their patient and ensure that the physicians of Lima "are treated with the decorum they merit" (7). This time, however, Dorotea was ready for a fight, and so were her many followers. Rather than waiting to be arrested, Dorotea presented herself to the authorities and invoked the protection of the "Supreme Government" on the basis that her right to a fair prosecution had been violated, since those accusing her were also the main witnesses to her alleged crime (8–9). She depicted herself as "an old and helpless woman" who was persecuted by a powerful and illegitimate institution for curing those unfortunate souls who insistently begged her for help (8). She characterized her actions as a "deed of charity and a matter of religion," and said it would be a great offence to God to abandon her patients to their fate, knowing that she had in her hands the power to save them. As for her remedies, Dorotea insisted that they were nothing more than a few well-chosen herbs. She charged only what she had spent on buying them; and for those who were unable to pay, she gave them free of charge. Unmoved by her arguments, the Protomedicato and the doctors who had brought the case against her demanded that she be punished according to a royal decree dated 21 November 1733, in which Phillip V had sentenced those who practised medicine lacking proper authorization to a hefty fine and banishment from the city. According to Valdés and his colleagues, the decree was still in effect and was legally binding, since the new republican authorities had not repealed the laws regulating the office of the Protomedicato, as they had with some other colonial legislation, because these laws did not contradict the constitution and the fundamental principles of the republic (10).

Phillip V's decree had indeed not been repealed, but it was an ill-advised move to invoke a law promulgated by a Spanish king in order to punish a popular folk healer. Almost immediately after her second arrest and the beginning of her trial early in 1831, a growing number of citizens – and not exclusively from Lima's lower classes – began to voice their support for the *curandera*. One of the first shots fired in what would become a prolonged battle over the boundaries of medicine, politics, and individual freedoms in Peru appeared in the *Mercurio peruano*. In February 1831, a concerned citizen submitted an anonymous letter criticizing the various forms of legal harassment suffered by Dorotea and questioning the true motives of the Protomedicato. In this regard, he suggested that Valdés, Tafur, and other doctors wanted to get rid of Dorotea not because her methods were unscientific but because of her surprising rate of success. In fact, he argued, she was able to cure her patients rapidly and at little expense thanks to "the simple use of some herbs with which Nature has provided her" (*Mercurio peruano*, 16 February 1831, 4). After alerting the public to the fact that no less than eighteen depositions from the most respected citizens had been collected to support Dorotea during her trial, he concluded by affirming that it was the Protomedicato and not Dorotea that needed to be banned from the republic. As he put it,

Ten years have passed since we achieved our independence. Ever since then, and with this sacred idea in mind, we have endured every form of sacrifice in order to remove from our country all forms of fanaticism, arbitrariness, and despotism. It is therefore unthinkable for us Peruvians that in the land of the free, there can still be a feudal tribunal such as the office of the Protomedicato, which has despotically persecuted an unhappy woman, the mother of many children, whose only fault is to resurrect those who die at the hands of the protomédico and his colleagues. (Ibid.)

The Protomedicato reacted swiftly. Just two days after the publication of the letter, the *Mercurio peruano* printed a brief response submitted under the pseudonym "Svadel," the pen name that Valdés had used in his contributions to the first *Mercurio peruano*. In it, he scoffed at Dorotea's miraculous healing abilities and heroic virtues, which he described as consisting of her willingness "to inject patients with unsalted lard, charge 20 reales for each enema, and receive one peso for each visit" (*Mercurio peruano*, 18 February 1831, 1). As for the large number of citizens who allegedly endorsed Dorotea's methods, Valdés asked whether someone had taken the time to count those whom she had killed with her remedies and provided several examples of the treatment's harmful effects. Peruvian medicine, he averred, as practised by licensed doctors and supervised by the Protomedicato, was the same scientific medicine taught and practised throughout the civilized world. To defend it from "the many charlatans who wish to become physicians" was the duty not only of the protomédico but of all citizens of Lima (ibid., 2). According to Valdés, nobody should defend tricksters such as Dorotea on the basis of protecting the individual freedoms upheld in the constitution. Otherwise, he predicted, those rights would degenerate, and "in a short time, Lima will be known not as the city of the free but of the barbarians" (ibid.).

Valdés's letter did not appease the supporters of Dorotea. On the contrary, it incensed them even further. The first response was published a few days later. It refuted all the cases that Valdés had cited as evidence against her and praised the folk healer for discovering the beneficial effects of many natural remedies while criticizing the pedantry of doctors (*Mercurio peruano*, 22 February 1831, 4). Three days later, a certain Miguel Blanco – one of Dorotea's patients mentioned by Valdés – felt compelled to write an open letter signed with his own name declaring that Valdés's account was an unfaithful representation of the facts. Blanco attributed his recovery to the almost miraculous remedies prescribed by Dorotea and not to the many bloodlettings that had been ordered by his doctors (*Mercurio peruano*, 25 February 1831, 3).[3] Even less sympathetic towards the Protomedicato was a letter that appeared in the *Mercurio peruano* the following day, written by someone who identified himself simply as *un consejero imparcial* (an impartial observer). After disclosing that he was neither a doctor nor a patient of Dorotea, he resolutely affirmed that if the occasion required it, he would most certainly place his health in the hands of the *curandera*. He noted in particular her record of succesful cures and the lower cost of her remedies and medical visits compared with that of regular medicine and licensed physicians. As for the number of patients allegedly killed by Dorotea, the author asked Valdés to estimate how many had died as a result of doctors' negligence and reasoned that if Dorotea had killed six for every thousand she had saved, "doctors have probably saved six for every thousand they have killed" (*Mercurio peruano*, 26 February 1831, 2). Finally, he posed a simple yet fundamental question: "If I am responsible for my own health, should I not be allowed to choose who should treat me and how? Of course, I should" (ibid.).

This was also the argument used two days later by an author who signed as "the Anti-Svadel" and questioned the very existence of the Protomedicato in early republican Peru. The Anti-Svadel asked his fellow citizens whether, in light of the actions taken by the Protomedicato, Peruvians could really be considered free of tyranny in their own country. The answer was a resounding "no." The office headed by Tafur was nothing more than a relic of the past, he asserted. He considered it incompatible with the constitutional principles of "*liberty* – since it gives access to knowledge exclusively to a specific group of men; *equality* – because it perpetuates the privileges of an extremely pernicious medical aristocracy; *individual security* – on account of its use of penal law to threaten citizens and reinforce class differences; and *property* – by oppressing industry and restricting profits to the members of the medical establishment" (*Mercurio peruano*, 28 February 1831, 3).[4] The Anti-Svadel claimed that far from contributing to the advancement of medicine, the Protomedicato had always been a formidable obstacle to its progress. It was unnecessary even from an administrative point of view since, in his opinion, the certification of surgeons and physicians could be done more easily, faster, and with less expense if universities and professional colleges were to assume its functions.

The Anti-Svadel's letter was probably the straw that broke the camel's back. On 3 March 1831, an angry José Manuel Valdés submitted a long and defiant letter to the *Mercurio peruano*. Again using the pseudonym Svadel, Valdés justified the persecution of Dorotea Salguero on both scientific and legal grounds. He maintained that all civilized nations of the world had erected laws against folk healers in order to protect reason, justice, and the common good. Doctors were granted exclusive rights to cure the sick because they had passed the most demanding exams, had devoted their lives to the scientific study of the human body, and had learned to compare their own observations with those of their predecessors. Keeping the disciplines of pharmacy and medicine separate – a separation that Dorotea challenged – was a key safeguard put in place to protect patients from the "sordid interest" of monetary gain by doctors who might otherwise prescribe unnecessary medicines (*Mercurio peruano*, 3 March 1831, 2). If the laws that protected the status quo in medical practice were removed and institutions such as the Protomedicato abolished, nothing would prevent folk healers from doing as they pleased, causing all sorts of problems for the republic. In those circumstances, predicted Valdés, it would require the lives and fortunes of many citizens before the public would be able to distinguish between good practitioners and impostors. But even after the division had been established, tricksters would only need to move to a new city in order to continue committing their "legal murders."[5]

Fortunately, Perú had not yet become such a barbarous country, added Valdés, and he judged it unlikely that the Anti-Svadel's proposals would become law anytime soon. Indeed, he was strongly convinced that medicine would always be cultivated and taught in Lima as a profession of the utmost importance to society and that the office of the Protomedicato would always be in charge of its supervision. In a heartfelt defence of his colleague Miguel Tafur, he added that if the protomédico were no longer to be entrusted with that task, he would be relieved of a responsibility that "does not provide any advantage or glory and that, on the contrary, exposes him to unjust claims from men who offend his gentleness without consideration of his experience, his decency, his deep knowledge, and his long-standing and untarnished reputation" (*Mercurio peruano*, ibid., 2 fn). But if, despite everything, the public still believes that Dorotea should be allowed to continue practising, wrote Valdés, the only alternative will be

> to revoke the licences of physicians so that no one will have to entrust his life to these ignorant murderers when there is a *doctora* who possesses the skills to cure him. It will also be essential to prohibit the study of anatomy, physiology, pathology, etc., since they will not be necessary to becoming a good doctor. The authorities should entrust her with a hospital so that patients receive the incomparable benefit of being cured by her wisdom and students may learn from her extraordinary knowledge. To honour her memory, the nation should hang paintings in the Colegio de medicina, in the university and in the auditorium where clinical medicine is taught. These paintings will depict the Temple of Asclepius and the god of medicine himself leading Dorotea to a magnificent throne and placing his snake-entwined staff in her hands. The nymphs of the Rimac will crown her head with a garland made not of laurel – like that of the son of Apollo – but of the herbs from which she prepares her miraculous remedies. Hippocrates, Galen, Sydenham, and Boerhaave will be at her feet, serving as her footstool. And to express the humiliation of these princes of medicine and the triumph of the new goddess, the following inscription will be engraved in gold letters: SHE SURPASSED THEM WITHOUT DOCTRINE, WITHOUT BOOKS, AND WITHOUT TEACHERS. (*Mercurio peruano*, 3 March 1831, 3)

Valdés's article did not stop letters in support of Dorotea Salguero from continuing to appear in the *Mercurio peruano*.[6] The biggest shock to those who defended the Protomedicato, however, came on 2 April 1831, when the verdict of her trial was announced. Contrary to Valdés's and Tafur's expectations, the judge ruled that the prosecution had not proved that Dorotea Salguero killed anyone with her remedies. The judge supported the defendant's claims that those she treated were considered beyond any hope of recovery by their own doctors and had therefore nothing to lose. He based his conclusions on the testimony of seventeen witnesses of an "exceptional" and "trustworthy" reputation (*Defensa* 1831, 48). As for the charge of practising medicine without a licence and deceiving her patients into believing that she was a true doctor, the tribunal ruled that Dorotea had never claimed to be a professional physician, even though people commonly referred to her as *la doctora*. Far from condemning her, the tribunal recognized Dorotea's actions as having been motivated by Christian compassion for her fellow men, and it reaffirmed her right to prepare, sell, and administer herbal remedies whose harvest and consumption "are not forbidden to anybody" (44–5).

As for the Protomedicato, the verdict strongly criticized the conception of medicine that Tafur and Valdés defended. The tribunal cited the opinion of several modern scholars – including some university professors in Lima – who considered medicine "an art as fallible and diverse as human nature" and disputed its status as a science on account of its lack of "firm principles from which to draw true demonstrations" (45). Echoing the arguments of Dorotea's liberal allies, the tribunal also questioned the legality of invoking a decree that was part of a "defective and mutilated legal code unable to govern a free nation," and it resolutely affirmed that no law could force free men to have their ailments cured exclusively by certified physicians (45–6); citizens should be free to choose, since "nobody has a greater interest in his own life than he who is at imminent risk of losing it" (49). Based on these considerations, the tribunal ruled that Dorotea Salguero should not be bothered or persecuted by the Protomedicato, although it asked Congress to clarify the "various and grave points of doubt that frequently arise in this kind of trial" (49).[7]

Unsurprisingly, the voices that advocated the dissolution of the Protomedicato grew louder after the Dorotea Salguero affair, and they became even more so following the death of Miguel Tafur on 7 December 1833 (Lastres 1943, xix). Less than a week after his passing, a newspaper article appeared with the title "No más Protomedicato" [No more Protomedicato] (*Mercurio peruano*, 13 December 1833, 2). Signing simply as "someone who cares for the good of his country," the author argued that Tafur's death offered the chance to replace the Protomedicato with a *junta* made of six or seven university professors – to be known as the Facultad de Medicina – who would assume the responsibilities of that office. Among other shortcomings, the text accused the Protomedicato not just of being an obsolete institution but also of having failed to achieve the goal of placing Peruvian medicine on a par with that practised in the most-developed countries in Europe by perpetuating outmoded medical theories. The Protomedicato's harmful influence was particularly noticeable in the dreadful state of the Colegio de la Independencia, which, according to the author of the article, had not made a single step forward since its inauguration. In order to reverse this situation, he advocated using the funds traditionally allocated to the Protomedicato to increase the budget of the school and the number of its faculty members. With new funds and under the supervision of the new *junta*, the Colegio de la Independencia could finally serve the purpose for which it had been conceived. Classes and demonstrations could again be offered on a regular basis. Students would no longer have to study without proper supervision or be left to select on their own the most appropriate books for each subject. Guided by "enlightened and experienced professors," they would learn "the true principles of the medical sciences from the book of nature itself" (ibid.). It was indeed possible, concluded the author, to build a new school from the ruins of the old one and allow future generations of Peruvian physicians to reach their full potential. There was but one condition: it was necessary "to start first by eradicating the Protomedicato" (ibid.).

The author of "No más Protomedicato" did not have to wait long for a reply. Just five days later, a group that identified itself simply as *Los amigos de su país* (the friends of the country) submitted a text to the same newspaper denouncing "his excessive ambitions." It is unknown whether Valdés or Gastañeta – who had replaced Tafur as protomédico – were among those who wrote the letter, but they must have shared the ideas put forward by the members of that group. *Los amigos de su país* started by denouncing the aforementioned article as the work of a foreigner who had no other objective than to advance his own career "by injuring the well-deserved reputation of Peruvian doctors and reforming the institutions of a country in which he was not born" (*Mercurio peruano* 18 December 1833, 3). They subsequently dismissed his proposal for establishing a *junta* by arguing that such an institution – the Junta de sanidad – already existed in Peru as a counterweight to the powers of the Protomedicato.[8] As for his opinion about the Colegio de la Independencia, they considered it "a lie and an insult" to suggest that its students had to learn medicine on their own because of a lack of capable instructors. On the contrary, ever since Hipólito Unanue had founded it, the school had been characterized by the quality of its faculty and its engagement with the latest medical theories. Much of the school's success was due to the efforts of Miguel Tafur, who had done everything in his power as protomédico to keep the school running "in spite of the difficulties that the school had suffered as a result of the scarcity of revenue" (ibid.). *Los amigos de su país* attributed the alleged falsehoods contained in "No más Protomedicato" to personal animosities and professional rivalries. Therefore, they recommended the newspaper's readers to ignore the suggestions made by this author and to treat his insults to Peruvian professors "with the utmost disdain, since they had been motivated by the darkest envy" (ibid., 4).

It was not until 1835, when Felipe Salaverry gained power and Valdés became Protomédico general de la República that the Peruvian government finally sided with those who supported the thesis of the Protomedicato. On 3 April of that year, General Salaverry restored to the Protomedicato the authority to oversee pharmacies and medicines, a responsibility it had lost in 1831 (*Colección de leyes* 1862 [1835], vol. 9, 86; see also *Índice general* 1845, 674). Three days later, he enlarged these powers by issuing a decree that granted the chief medical office the powers it had had at the beginning of the republican era. Salaverry based his decision on the fact that the laws passed since then to reform the Peruvian health system – which had the effect of curtailing the authority of the protomédico – had encountered in practice "a thousand inconveniences not foreseen by legislators" (*Colección de leyes* 1862 [1835], vol. 9, 86). The decree also recognized the "urgent necessity of closing the door to charlatans of both genders, who had taken advantage of the criminal tolerance shown by authorities to earn a living off the destruction of humanity" (ibid.). The laws promulgated by Salaverry made Valdés the most powerful protomédico since Hipólito Unanue, and Valdés did not hesitate to use these powers in order to impose his own conception of medicine and the authority of the Protomedicato on Lima's medical profession. His resolve, however, was soon tested by a proud representative of those who considered themselves at the forefront of Western medicine: a British physician named Archibald Smith.

Science and Nationalism

Among the first actions taken by Valdés as protomédico was a partial ban on the use of calomel in the treatment of dysentery, a disease that accounted for about 15 percent of all deaths in Lima by the late 1830s (Bustios Romani 2004, 242). Valdés restricted the use of calomel, a mercury compound, because of the many problems that "its untimely administration and scandalous abuse" caused in the city. Lima's physicians would be allowed to administer the substance only under the direct supervision of one of the Protomedicato's doctors, who would charge a fee of four reales in return for his services. Valdés threatened to suspend the medical licences of those who failed to comply with the new regulation (*El Rejenerador*, 2 June 1835, 2). In order to legitimize his decree, Valdés cited the recent publication of a study on dysentery that had established "the means by which we should combat this disease that is rampant in our country according to the extensive experience of its author and the authority of the profession's most respected practitioners" (ibid.). The text was entitled *Memoria sobre la disentería, sus causas, prognóstico y curación*, and the author was none other than José Manuel Valdés. For those few readers who were still unaware, the book's title page reminded them of the great influence and prestige that Valdés had accumulated in Peruvian medicine in the years following the country's independence. In addition to his position as Protomédico general de la República, Valdés held the titles of Catedrático de Prima de medicina at the Universidad de San Marcos, director of the Colegio de la Independencia de Lima, and member of Madrid's Royal Academy of Medicine. His aim in writing the report was to explain why dysentery had become much more common in Lima than in the past and why, being of a more benign variety than the dysentery commonly experienced in Europe, it had resulted in a noticeable increase in the mortality rate among those suffering from it in the city (Valdés 1835a, 7). Even though he conceded that political and natural causes may have played an important role,[9] he ultimately blamed inadequate care as the main culprit.

According to Valdés, many in Lima preferred to use home remedies instead of relying on doctors' treatments, particularly when the latter involved bloodletting, which he considered an appropriate therapy in nearly every case of dysentery (ibid., 9). Others turned to the many folk healers still active in Lima who promised to cure dysentery, along with a wide array of other illnesses, for a fraction of the cost charged by doctors and pharmacists. But since neither home remedies nor folk healers were particularly new phenomena, Valdés reasoned that the explanation for the increased number of deaths from dysentery might lie elsewhere. Calomel, for Valdés, was the prime suspect, since it was one of the "remedies" that made even the most benign dysentery lethal (ibid., 11). English physicians and their followers, who were influential in early republican Peru, had popularized its use as a treatment for this disease. Encouraged by the success with which it had been employed in the British possessions in India and guided by what Valdés labelled a "blind empiricism," English doctors had imprudently generalized its use to the treatment of all kinds of fever "without consideration of the type of fever or any other circumstances" (ibid.). Valdés even suggested that in recommending calomel as a remedy for dysentery, these doctors were not guided by scientific reasoning – since they lacked a clear understanding of why mercurial preparations were an effective treatment against the disease – but were influenced by foreign commercial interests, since the calomel used in Lima had to be imported and was not subject to the Protomedicato's inspection (Valdés 1835a, 13–14).

Valdés became even more suspicious after he discovered that the adverse secondary effects of calomel had already been denounced by the president of the British Medico-Botanical Society, Earl Stanhope. In a speech given on 16 January 1830, Stanhope had urged doctors and botanists to find a vegetal substance that could replace the compound (Stanhope 1830, 29). According to Valdés, his warning was echoed in the works of the most respected doctors in Europe: "Zimmerman and Stoll in Germany, Carminati y Burserio in Italy, Pinera in Spain, the school of Montpellier and of Leon, and the most distinguished physicians of Paris, Bosquillon, Pinel, Alibert, Broussais *et alia*" (Valdés 1835a, 13–14). Valdés believed it was time for Peruvian doctors to follow in the footsteps of these leading physicians and begin curing dysentery according to the methods best suited to the Peruvian context and not according to those suggested by the British physicians who resided in Lima.

Just two days after the publication of Valdés's decree, an anonymous letter appeared in *El Rejenerador* accusing the protomédico and his allies of having orchestrated a "master-stroke" in order to establish "the monopoly of monopolies" with nothing but their own interests in mind. The letter charged Valdés with both arrogance (for believing he was the only physician who knew how to cure dysentery) and ignorance (for basing his conclusions on outdated science and imposing his own scientific judgment over those of British doctors) (*El Rejenerador*, 9 June 1835, 2). Valdés showed little patience with this and similar challenges to his decision. In a reply signed with his name, he called his opponents "stupid" and "ignorant." Moreover, he threatened to re-examine all those doctors and surgeons who, in the opinion of the Protomedicato, were guilty of "grave" and "frequent" mistakes in the treatment of patients. He also announced that those who resisted the re-examination would have their medical licences suspended, while those who failed the exam would have their names placed on a public list (*El Rejenerador*, 16 June 1835, 1–2). He justified his authority to do so by referring to the decrees that had restored to the Protomedicato the jurisdiction and status granted in the old colonial legislation, of which it had been robbed by "a misguided and ill-fated liberalism" (ibid.). He also published a letter of appreciation by a patient who thanked him for "having spared me from becoming a victim of calomel, which was prescribed to me by Dr D. Juan Salazar and the other physicians of his medical *junta*" (ibid.).[10]

Valdés's threats were not to be taken lightly. Three days later, the said Juan de Dios Salazar published a text in which he accused Valdés of personal animosity, as well as criticizing him for issuing "a general condemnation against all those who, deviating from his doctrines, make use of calomel in the treatment of dysentery" (*El Rejenerador*, 19 June 1835, 2). He denounced the protomédico for trying to replace a trusted remedy with his own – based on "bloodletting left, right, and centre" – and for scandalously invoking colonial laws that were in opposition to the country's freedoms and constitutional guarantees. If the government had restored to the Protomedicato the powers it had in 1821, Salazar argued, it was only "to correct abuses and not to carry out personal vengeance" (ibid.). As for the threat of re-examination, he challenged Valdés to participate in a joint examination at which an independent tribunal would decide which of the two was the better doctor.

This time, Valdés did not need to answer his critic directly. Someone who used the penname Lanzarote took up his defence in a sarcastic letter that appeared a few days later in *El Rejenerador*. Lanzarote suggested that Salazar voluntarily submit himself for re-examination so that the doubts about his suitability for the practice of medicine could be dispelled. If he passed, Lanzarote ironically told Salazar, "I will invite my friends and a group of young people to celebrate your triumph at the door of the tribunal with noisemakers and fireworks" (*El Rejenerador*, 26 June 1835, 1–2). The whole issue degenerated into absurdity when, two days later, a contributor to *El Rejenerador*, who signed simply as Tomé, called Lanzarote the "proto-cocinero de Galeno" (Galen's proto-cook) (*El Rejenerador*, 28 June 1835, 2); shortly afterwards, someone who identified himself as Bachiller Sansón Carrasco – a reference to one of the characters of Cervantes' novel *Don Quijote* – labelled him a "mellow doctor," "phlebotomist ad partem," and "protomédico ad extra," as well as other demeaning names (*El Rejenerador*, 3 July 1835, 1–2). But then the controversy suddenly took a more serious turn, revealing how close Valdés was to causing a diplomatic incident.

This occurred when *El Rejenerador* published a special supplement that included the text of a letter of complaint that a doctor named Archibald Smith had written to the British consul in Lima, which the consul had sent to the British Foreign Office in London.[11] Smith had complained that the protomédico's decision deprived the city's doctors of their own medical judgment and reduced experienced physicians to the role of mere tools in "a system devised by Dr Valdés" (*El Rejenerador*, supplt., 19 July 1835, 1). Smith's observations at the Hospital de Santa Ana had convinced him that the protomédico's approach was fundamentally wrong and that calomel was "an essential remedy," without which it was not possible to treat the illness effectively. Moreover, he accused Valdés – who also had worked at Santa Ana – of causing innumerable deaths with his treatments (ibid.).[12] Smith also informed the consul that the British Treasury would have to cover the fees demanded by the Protomedicato every time a British doctor deemed it necessary to administer calomel. Even in such cases, no doctor could be sure of being authorized to use it, given the arbitrariness of the protomédico's decisions. In view of these circumstances, Smith concluded that he could no longer be held responsible for the lives of the British and American patients under his care. The British consul responded by sending an angry letter to the Foreign Office in London, in which he emphasized the unjustified nature of the ban and the clearly anti-British sentiments expressed by the Peruvian protomédico in his *Memoria sobre la disentería*. He argued that British patients should not be asked to trust the medical judgment of an individual whom "they know only by the notoriety of the slander that he has disseminated against our country's physicians and our national character" (*El Rejenerador*, supplt., 19 July 1835, 2). Therefore, he pleaded with the authorities in London to intervene so that British citizens, sailors, and doctors would be exempt from the protomédico's orders relating to the use of calomel and so that national honour could be restored. In the meantime, the consul made Valdés directly responsible for any British lives lost as a result of his mandate (ibid.).

Valdés did his best to contain the situation and avoid what could rapidly become a serious incident that might jeopardize his career. In a letter written to the Peruvian Foreign Office, he clarified that doctors working in hospitals were not included in his prohibition to use calomel, which extended only to those who administered it as part of their private practice. This meant that Smith, who attended to his patients at the Hospital de Santa Ana, had been exempt from the prohibition all along. Valdés made Dr Fuentes, another member of the Protomedicato, accountable for what he considered to be nothing more than a case of miscommunication. Since both Fuentes and Smith worked in the same hospital, Valdés had assumed that Fuentes would have already informed his British colleague of the details. Nevertheless, Valdés also placed some of the blame on Archibald Smith, who could have raised the issue with Fuentes before taking up his complaint with the British consul and, as a result, distracting the Peruvian government at a time of great political strife (ibid.). The British consul accepted the explanations provided by Valdés and the Peruvian Foreign Office. He then wrote to Archibald Smith informing him that he was exempt from the Protomedicato's prohibition, unbraiding him for not having consulted his colleagues before submitting his initial complaint (ibid., 3). With a somewhat injured sense of pride and angry at what he considered a tactical retreat by the protomédico, Smith denied that such an exemption had ever been made and that the ban would have remained in place if the British authorities had not taken any action in the matter (ibid.).

The whole issue could have stopped there had it not been for Smith's decision to publish, two days later, a long article publicly attacking the medical opinions expressed by Valdés in his *Memoria sobre la disentería*. Smith once again praised the beneficial effects of mercurial preparations in general, which he attributed to their ability to act on the circulatory system, the liver, and the intestines in a more effective manner than any other known medicine. Used appropriately and diligently, Smith argued, calomel was as safe as the best medicine, and he cited as proof not only his own experience with it but also that of Sydenham, whose views on the matter "have more weight for an enlightened soul than a whole book full of rhetoric and purely speculative arguments" (*El Rejenerador*, supplt., 21 July 1835, 1). Smith also accused Valdés of misrepresenting the words of Earl Stanhope, the president of the British Medico-Botanical Society. According to Smith, Stanhope had simply expressed his desire that botanists should find a substitute for calomel, which they had not yet done; he had never argued that it should be abandoned immediately. As for the physicians cited by Valdés to support his views, most of them were already dead by the time James Johnson published his authoritative work *The Influence of Tropical Climates on European Constitutions* (1813), in which the effectiveness of calomel and its utility in the treatment of dysentery was established once and for all (ibid., 2).[13]

For Smith, it was not just Valdés's opinions on dysentery that were wrong, it was his entire conception of medicine. He challenged Valdés's assertion that the remedies used to treat a specific illness had to be tailored to the illness's native region or to the specific "constitutions" of that region's inhabitants. People were basically identical in all parts of the globe. This being the case, Smith had no doubt that "calomel cures dysentery among Peruvians in Peru no less effectively than among the English in India" (ibid.). The work of a physician was for him not unlike that of an astronomer: the latter sought to uncover the general and universal laws that ruled the cosmos, whereas the former aspired to do the same for that "delicate but well-balanced system of flesh and blood" that was the human body. In order for medicine to become a rigorous science, its remedies should conform "to the common and invariable laws of animal economy." The patient's accidental circumstances – his place of birth or residence, the strength or weakness of his temperament, his diet and habits, etc. – should merely act as the terrain that every able doctor, no matter where he is, "must be able to interpret at a single glance, just as a military tactician does on a new battlefield" (ibid.). Not only was Valdés's conception of medicine *passé*, but it was based on a xenophobic animosity to British science, as demonstrated by the protomédico's groundless accusation that English doctors were "empiricists." Smith claimed that no country had rewarded scientific and literary endeavours better or produced better scientists and men of letters than England. He reminded Valdés that "knowledge is the source of power" and that England had "always cultivated the former in order to secure the latter" (ibid., 1). The difference in the political and scientific standing of the two countries, Smith believed, could not be more dramatic.

Valdés reacted furiously to what he saw as an attack not just on himself but on Peruvian medicine and the country in general. In a pamphlet entitled *Al público peruano*, Valdés denounced Smith's "scandalous text" as being born of envy rather than scientific zeal, and he named the cause of Smith's animosity. Hostilitiy between the two had begun a few years earlier over a difference of opinion during the treatment of several high-profile patients. As was common in these cases, medical decisions were made by a *junta* made up four or five of the city's most distinguished physicians. Valdés and Smith had worked together in such *juntas* on at least three separate occasions. Each time, the majority of the *junta* had decided to follow Valdés's recommendations rather than those of Smith, a fact that the British doctor deeply resented.[14] However, Valdés insisted that his prohibition against calomel had nothing to do with these disagreements. Once again, he stressed that the ban had been issued in order to prevent the abuses that "some ignorant and stubborn physicians" committed in their private practice (Valdés 1835b, 3); and he repeated that doctors serving in hospitals or those in charge of foreign citizens were not included in the ban (4). As for Smith's implication that, for personal gain, the protomédico charged a fee to supervise the use of calomel, Valdés not only denied it but accused Smith of hypocrisy, since doctors in Britain charged far more and more frequently for similar services (5). Had he wished to get rich supervising the use of calomel in the treatment of dysentery, he would not have prohibited it.

Valdés also challenged Smith to produce the name of even one doctor from a nation other than Britain who supported his "imaginary theory that has sent many to the sepulchre" (Valdés 1835b, 11). Valdés categorically denied that his opinions had anything to do with patriotism but said he could not remain indifferent when a foreigner like Smith demeaned Peruvian science and pretended "to know the illnesses of Peru better than the likes of Bueno, Aguirre, Moreno, and Tafur" (6). It was absurd to forget their contributions and to equate, as Smith had done, the laws of physiology with those of physics (27). Doctors were not astronomers, since "astronomers are able to calculate with precision the movement and positions of the planets as they orbit their star, whereas doctors, with nothing more than obscure and equivocal symptoms to guide them into the sanctuary of nature, usually cannot determine which organ is affected and, as a result, fail to prescribe the appropriate remedies" (27–8). Moreover, inspired by Baglivio, Valdés argued that it was necessary to treat illnesses in a different manner according to the atmosphere and customs of each nation. From it, he inferred the corollary that "foreign physicians should always consult with experienced local doctors in the countries in which they establish themselves, asking about the most frequent illnesses, their causes, varieties, irregularities, and possible treatment" (28). Reviving one of Tafur's proposals, Valdés concluded by strongly advocating the creation of a "code of Peruvian medicine" to guide those establishing their practice in Peru, a project that he had not ceased to promote among his illustrious colleagues (29).

In order to put an end to the controversy and avoid another diplomatic incident at a time of particular political instability, the government of Felipe Santiago de Salaverry made a Solomonic decision. It declared the Protomedicato's ban on the use of calomel void but affirmed its authority to re-examine any Peruvian doctors "whose ineptitude caused formal complaints to be submitted in writing" (*El Rejenerador*, supplt., 29 September 1835, 2; *Colección de leyes, decretos y órdenes* 1862, 9: 138–9). The government chose not to judge the scientific merits of the two antagonists' opposing views on the treatment of dysentery and on medicine in general. It simply ruled that once a doctor had passed the medical exams, it was "insulting to his honour to restrict him from administering those remedies that he deemed suitable in each case" (ibid.). Valdés probably thought that Salaverry's decision undermined his authority, but he had no choice but to comply.

As for Smith, he returned to England a few months later, where he wrote a book detailing his experience in Peru that he entitled *Peru as*

It Is. As was to be expected, Smith panned nearly every aspect of the teaching and practice of medicine in Peru. He derided the climatic theories that enabled Peruvian doctors to dismiss the validity of foreign medical opinions by simply claiming that "he does not know our climate." Mockingly, Smith speculated that perhaps there really was "something occult in the climate of Lima, which only a Limenian or Creole physician can sufficiently comprehend" (Smith 1839, 46). He once again expressed his conviction that the laws of physiology, like any other natural law, were the same in Peru as in England and that, consequently, medical treatments should be similar in all parts of the world (ibid., 49–50). As for the infamous medical *juntas* that Valdés had referred to in his defence, Smith dismissed them as "remarkable occasions of oratorical display" in which "the warmest discussion frequently turns on the dose, composition, or medicinal operation of some common drug; and all the learning, method, and criticism, sometimes discovered at these solemn debates, terminate not unfrequently in the most simple practice, by which the nurse is enjoined to have recourse to the *jeringa*, and the patient told he must drink *agua de pollo*, or chicken-tea, until the return of the *junta*" (ibid., 97–8).[15]

Death of a Protomédico

The controversy with Archibald Smith did not dampen Valdés's enthusiasm for scientific pursuits nor does it seem to have done permanent damage to his reputation. In fact, Andrés de Santa Cruz – who replaced Salaverry as the ruler of Peru in 1836 – awarded Valdés the medal of the national Legion of Honour in recognition of his many achievements (Lavalle n.d., 19). A letter acknowledging receipt by the Royal Academy of Medicine in Paris of two of Valdés's essays – one of them being *Al público peruano* – was exhibited in one of Lima's pharmacies as if it were the ultimate proof of the triumph of his ideas – and of Peruvian medicine in general – over those of English physicians (Herrera 1843, 3). Science and writing also found a place in Valdés's daily activities as protomédico. Following the government's request that he determine the best course of action to prevent the possible spread of *colera morbus* in Lima, Valdés published in 1838 a treatise in which he compared the "sporadic" outbreaks of cholera observed in the capital of Peru with the "epidemic" variety that "has wreaked such havoc in both the Old and New Worlds" (Valdés 1838, 2; *Colección de leyes* 1862 [1837], 8: 340).

Meanwhile, the protomédico's strained relationship with foreign doctors continued. In 1838 an Italian physician named José Indelicato begged for the Peruvian government's protection against "the constant and cruel persecution" he was suffering at the hands of Juan de Gastañeta, one of Valdés's main assistants and a former protomédico (*Reclamo* 1838, 2). Indelicato had been forced to pay the maximum licensing fees for practising medicine in Lima, despite his recent arrival in the city and his lack of patients. He tried to leave the country, but because of his debts, he was arrested and his passport withheld before he could do so. Gastañeta justified charging maximum fees to foreign doctors on protectionist and nationalist grounds. He argued that foreign doctors were not entitled to the same benefits as their Peruvian counterparts, especially since the fees that foreign doctors charged for their services where often much higher. Gastañeta mantained that they were able to charge more thanks to the taste for novelty of Lima's ruling class and the fact that foreigners, who were usually wealthier, preferred to employ their countrymen rather than Peruvians (ibid., 1–2). Peru's changing political situation also worked against other doctors who had considered themselves relatively safe from such harassment. On 8 March 1839, after the dissolution of the Peru-Bolivian Confederation, Valdés revoked the medical license of the Bolivian physician Juan Enrique Serivener, arguing that the legislation that had allowed him to practise medicine and surgery in Peru was no longer valid. Valdés threatened to have Serivener fined and punished if he continued to practise "without being re-examined and approved by the Protomedicato" (AGN, RAME, 839, 1, 110, 1 f).[16]

Despite Valdés's defence of their economic interests, a growing number of doctors resented his attempt to control their medical practice and faulted the Protomedicato for what they considered the sorry state of Peruvian medicine two decades after independence. Nothing exemplified this better than the alarming state in which the Colegio de la Independencia found itself. By the late 1830s it was evident – even to an ardent supporter of the school such as Valdés – that failed reforms, political instability, and a shortage of funds had left the school founded by Unanue, as well as Lima's health system, in a precarious position.

The Peruvian authorities had already substantially scaled back Unanue's original – and overly ambitious – plans for the college. Regulations enacted in 1826 had limited the "medical staff to one professor of anatomy, another of physiology, one in pathology, one for external and internal clinical work, one for therapy and pharmacy, and one for surgery and obstetrics" (*Colección de leyes* 1862 [1826], 9: 157–8). The cuts were supposed to remain in effect only until the country's financial and political situation improved, but persistent instability meant that any further development of medical institutions was put on hold. As a result, the school languished for most of the next two decades, in spite of the best efforts of its directors Miguel Tafur and Cayetano Heredia. The situation did not pass unnoticed by foreign travellers. The Swiss naturalist Johan Jakob von Tschudi, who spent four years in Peru in the late 1830s, blamed what he perceived as the lack of theoretical and clinical instruction in Peru on the weakness of the Colegio de la Independencia, a name "that it justly merits, for certainly medicine is taught there with a singular independence of all rules and systems." The situation at the school also helped to explain, he said, why many hospitals in Lima were so "lamentably defective in internal arrangement, and above all in judicious medical attendance" (Von Tschudi 1854, 49).

To remedy the situation, Agustín Gamarra, who succeeded Santa Cruz as president of Peru in 1839, appointed a *junta* to govern the college and gave Valdés a leading role (Lavalle [Zegarra] 26; Bustios Romani 2004, 295). The new *reglamento*, which was approved on 28 January 1840, placed the direction of the school back in the hands of the Protomédico general de la República (*Reglamento* 1862 [1840], título 2, art. 11). Day-to-day administrative and academic issues would, however, be the responsibility of a *rector* chosen by the civil authorities (ibid., título 3, art. 13). From an academic perspective, the curriculum was expanded, but it did not represent a radical departure from the way that medicine had been taught in Lima since the early nineteenth century. In addition to anatomy, physiology, and pathology, the new regulations called for instruction in hygiene, philosophy, clinical and practical medicine, pharmacy, surgery, midwifery, and topographical medicine. The regulations also established that "the theoretical part of medicine shall be taught by departmental heads in the anatomical amphitheatre or in the medical classrooms, whereas the practical part shall take place at the patients' bedsides and in the amphitheatre" and pharmacy should be studied "at the apothecary of nearby hospitals" (ibid., título 7, art. 32 and 33).[17] Despite representing an improvement, Valdés's reforms were short-lived. Juan Francisco de Vidal, who became president of Peru in 1842, returned Cayetano Heredia to the helm of the Colegio de la Independencia on 23 December of that year. Four months later, Heredia presented a new *reglamento* to replace the regulations that Valdés had established just three years earlier (*Colección de leyes* 1862 [1843], 9: 199–209). Valdés, whose health had already begun to deteriorate, did not dispute these changes – or at least he avoided doing so in public.[18]

Unfortunately, controversy followed Valdés to the end of his life. In June 1843 the newspaper *El Comercio* published statistics showing that 423 individuals had died during the month of May, a number well above average and an increase of 142 individuals compared with May 1842 (*El Comercio*, 1 June 1843, 2). The number caught the attention of the prefect of the Departmento de Lima, who two days later publicly requested that the protomédico offer a plausible explanation in order to "dispel the fear that yellow fever could reach Lima from Tumbez after having done so much damage in Guayaquil" (*El Comercio*, 3 June 1843, 2). Valdés's explanation did not deviate substantially from those he had previously offered concerning highly contagious illnesses. He attributed the high mortality rate to the fact that malignant fevers and epidemics had become more virulent and widespread because of environmental factors. He also blamed the sad state of Lima's hospitals and "the common misery brought about by civil unrest and repeated political upheavals" (*El Comercio*, 13 June 1843, 2). Valdés also decried the "empirical" methods employed by some doctors and the fact that everyone seemed to follow foreign rules instead of adopting the doctrine of the great practitioners of their own country: "some follow the example of the English, others the French, the Italians, the Germans, but very few practise *a la peruana*, that is, according to the principles of Peruvian medicine" (ibid.). The problem was aggravated by the shortage of trained physicians, the result of the decadence and lack of funds of the Colegio de la Independencia. Valdés clearly did not hold Heredia's recent reforms in high esteem since, in his opinion, the only way to improve public health was to "completely reform medical practice, which can only be achieved if the teaching of medicine is consis-

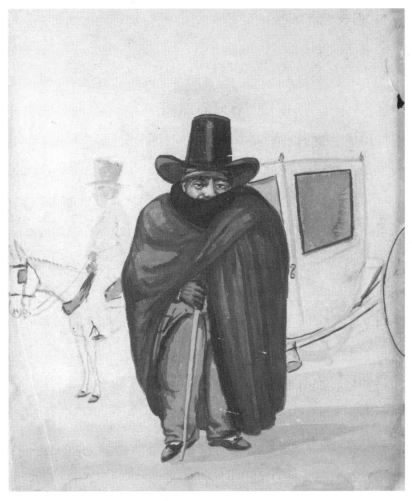

Doctor José Manuel Valdés, an Afro-Peruvian, rose to the top medical position in Peru in the 1830s.

tently carried out by enlightened doctors well versed in our country's climate and in its endemic and sporadic diseases" (ibid., 3). Only then, he claimed, will the Faculty of Medicine

recover its old splendour, which has been tarnished by ignorance and favouritism. The audacity of charlatans and folk healers, who con and murder the miserable patients whom they trick, will be repressed and punished; titles will only be granted to doctors who deserve them; no longer will professorships be granted to an internal candidate without fair competition; and the brilliant lectures of the past, those that merited the admiration and praise of men of letters, will again be heard in the university's auditoriums. Propelled by honour, students will immerse themselves in learning and, thanks to their achievements, their credit and reputation will depend not solely on the capriciousness of public opinion but on their own abilities; and professors will forever admire the fame that the school will acquire as a result of the efforts that, to this end, might be undertaken by Your Excellency, the wise and benefic Director who, under God's protection, so skilfully governs this Republic. (*El Comercio*, 13 June de 1843, 3)

Valdés's passionate but ultimately fruitless defence of his conception of Peruvian medicine was received with strong criticism. Three weeks after its appearance, *El Comercio* published the first of a series of anonymous texts that refuted his opinions, ridiculed his scientific standing, and questioned – as others had done years earlier – the very existence of the office of the Protomedicato. According to Lavalle, the articles were written by "a foreign charlatan, who having twice attempted to pass the medical exams, had failed on both occasions due to his total ignorance of the basic principles of the science he wished to practise and in spite of Valdés's benevolence and words of encouragement" (Lavalle [Zegarra] 30). Whether it was out of bitterness or conviction, the author of the articles directed a devastating critique of the colonial origins of the Protomedicato, calling it "an old shell from the unhappy time of the Austrian monarchs, a mouldy inquisitorial tribunal full of cobwebs, a corporation that smells of brotherhood, frozen in guilty inertia and with only the power to hurt" (*El Comercio*, 1 July 1843, 2).

The author also criticized the *ultra-peruanismo* (ultra-Peruvianism) of Valdés and labelled him "Medical Dictator of Peru" (*El Comercio*, 11 July 1843, 5). Hoisting the flag of progress, the author affirmed, as an undisputed fact, the existence of a "law of incessant and continual progress" governing the advancement of science, and said that it should be extended to medicine (*El Comercio*, 3 July 1843, 5). He considered it a serious mistake to proscribe the productions of human intellect merely because they had a foreign air, especially at a time when modern discoveries such as electricity, magnetism, and the Volt battery were opening the door to extraordinary changes: "If a new theory is wrong, it will decay and die; but if it is supported by reason and truth, nobody – not even the Protomédico de la República – will be able to stop it from becoming accepted by the masses" (*El Comercio*, 11 July 1843, 5). "The medical sciences in Peru," he declared, "should therefore adopt as their new paradigm not the one so cherished by Valdés but the one provided by Positivism, a fashionable word not yet included in the dictionary," that proposes that "nothing should be accepted without demonstration, exact reasoning, and positive evidence" (*El Comercio*, 17 July 1843, 7). The author concluded his attack on the Protomedicato by reminding Valdés that society demanded from doctors guarantees that his office could no longer provide. Instead of it, he proposed that a new medical society be founded on the basis of the aforementioned principles, which, "moved by the spirit of association and brotherhood, would promote benevolence, reciprocity, and mutual enlightenment among its members and would be protected from rivalry, envy, egoism, and private interests as a result" (ibid.).

Valdés did not have time to defend himself as he had done on so many occasions in the past: he died on 29 July 1843. His successor, José Dámaso Herrera, wrote a brief note – basically a eulogy – which he entitled "Servicios hechos a la medicina peruana por el doctor Valdés." Dámaso Herrera asserted that, with the exception of Valdés, "no other wise doctor who has lived in Peru since the times of the Spanish conquest had produced such a body of practical medical knowledge specific to this country based on their own observations and experience" (*El Comercio*, 13 July 1843, 3). Recognizing the solitude in which the protomédico found himself in the last years of his life, he lamented the fact that this fundamental contribution had yet to be recognized by many of his contemporaries. After summarizing some of the protomédico's other contributions, he praised Valdés for having reached the highest medical position in the republic in spite of his racial origins, and extolled him as an example "for those who were of the same or inferior castes" (ibid.). On 31 July 1843, just two days after the death of the protomédico, *El Comercio* joined Herrera in praising

Valdés. In its article "A la memoria del Dr. D.J. Manuel Valdés," the newspaper asserted that despite all criticisms,

> Dr Valdés rendered eminent services to his country, ennobling the name of Peru through his writings and giving it fame and esteem even among the learned nations of the Old Continent. As a citizen, he was obedient to the laws and a faithful observer of his social obligations. As a Christian, his entire life was a model of virtue and holiness: his profound wisdom was embellished by his moderation, his humility, his charity, and his piety. As a doctor, he possessed a most eminent knowledge of the field, and some of his medical treatises have been received by the luminaries of Europe with applause and admiration. (*El Comercio*, 31 July 1843, 4)

Science, Race, and Miracles

On 29 October 1837, Gregory XVI beatified the Dominican friar Martín de Porres in a solemn ceremony at the Vatican. News of his beatification filled Valdés with pride, but also with an intense sense of history. Martín de Porres had been the first mulatto to be widely respected by all social classes in Lima. His canonization process, which started immediately after his death, significantly improved the image of those of mixed African and European ancestry in the eyes of the colonial elite. On 27 February 1763, Pope Clement XIII declared his virtues to be heroic – a necessary step on the road to sainthood – and this too advanced the social standing of other members of his caste. As black medical practitioners, Larrinaga, Dávalos, and Valdés were heirs to a tradition that, for many, started in the humble infirmary of the Dominican friar. By the late 1830s, Dávalos and Larrinaga had already passed away, and an ageing Valdés was the last significant physician of African descent still active in the capital of Peru. Therefore, it was to a certain degree natural for the Dominican priest Lázaro Balaguer y Cubillas, chair of Theology at the University of San Marcos and one of the key figures behind Martin de Porres's beatification, to approach him with the request to write "a faithful account of the admirable life of this Limenean hero" (Valdés 1863 [1840], 5).[1]

Valdés asserted that his authority to write Martín de Porres's biography lay partly in the fact that both of them had "the same origins and shared the same humble birth" (ibid., 9). However, Valdés was also known in Lima as a gifted literary author who had written several religious books (ibid., 6). In 1818 he had published a small compilation of poems, translations, and commentaries on sacred subjects entitled *Poesías espirituales, escritas a beneficio y para el uso de las personas sencillas*, a work that he expanded in 1836. In 1822, as the Peruvian Constituent Congress debated – and rejected – the possibility of establishing freedom of religion in the new Republic, Valdés wrote La fe de Cristo triunfante en Lima, an ode to the "exceptional men" who, "making use of the powers granted by the people" had been able to defend the Catholic faith at a defining moment in the nation's history (Valdés 1822, 12–13).[2] In 1833 Valdés embarked on an even more ambitious literary project: an erudite translation and commentary on the Book of Psalms, *Salterio peruano*. Apart from its devotional purposes, the *Salterio* allowed Valdés to showcase his mastery of Latin and Spanish poetic meters. The book garnered the praise of the influential Spanish scholar Menéndez Pelayo, who considered it one of the best translations of the Psalms ever published in America, "due to the purity of its language and the simplicity and sweetness of its style, in which one can find echoes of Friar Luis de León's works" (Menéndez Pelayo 1948, 170). Valdés's qualities as a poet and as a lay theologian occupied as much space as his scientific achievements in the eulogy that *El Comercio* devoted to him in 1843. The panegyric praised the protomédico's deep knowledge of the Holy Scriptures and church doctrine and marvelled at his mastery of poetry, with which he was able to raise the spirits of his fellow men "up to the throne of the Divine Being" (*El Comercio*, 31 July 1843, 4).

Valdés saw the task entrusted to him by Father Balaguer y Cubillas as an opportunity to educate the public on the boundaries between medicine and religion. Like many of his contemporaries, Valdés rejected the existence of a rift between the two. He saw them as inextricably linked. The church had strongly influenced the practice of medicine in Peru since early colonial times, and it continued to do so, well into the nineteenth century. As early as 1550, Archbishop Loayza had reminded doctors of the important role that spiritual "medicines" should have in the care of patients admitted to the Hospital de Santa Ana, whose construction he had financed. He mandated that since many bodily illnesses begin as spiritual ones, all patients must confess their sins within twenty-four hours of their admission, "making them understand that the body can be healed more easily if one first heals the soul" (quoted in Lastres 1951a, 135). It was not only priests who emphasized the role of spiritual medicines in the treatment of patients. Doctors shared that opinion. José Miguel Ossera y Estella, chamber doctor for Viceroy Conde de la Monclova and himself a Peruvian protomédico, explored in his book *El físico cristiano* the sacred cures that should precede the treatment of any dangerous medical condition and insisted on the importance of devotional practices for a full physical and spiritual recovery (Ossera y Estella 1690, 1–8). Some priests also considered specialized medical and anatomical knowledge necessary in order to address the practical, moral, and theological dilemmas they encountered during their ministry. The best-known case was that of Francisco González Laguna, who in 1781 published *El zelo sacerdotal para con los niños no-nacidos*, in which he discussed the use of a caesarean section when a fetus was in danger of dying without receiving the Holy Sacraments.

The influence of religion in the practice of medicine in Peru was felt well into the nineteenth century. At the Colegio de medicina y cirugía de San Fernando – the most important scientific institution in late colonial Peru and the cornerstone of Unanue's project for medical reform – the doctors had agreed in 1816 to hold a mass daily, and they recognized the Virgin Mary as their patron three years later (Warren 2010, 210–11). Valdés himself believed that science – especially anatomy – could help fight atheism by revealing the infinite wisdom of the Creator: "Who does not marvel at the sight of this perfect machine made by the Almighty in which He combined the laws of hydraulics to propel the liquids through the vascular system, the laws of hydrostatic to explain their equilibrium, those of statics to create the levers, pulleys, and cords that animate its solid elements, and those of optics, catoptrics, and dioptrics to guide the direction, refraction, and reflection of light that allow our vision?" (Valdés 1792b, 180). Valdés's colleagues frequently indulged in similar thoughts. Miguel Tafur – Valdés's predecessor as head of the Protomedicato and one of the most relevant Limenean physicians in the first half of the nineteenth century – had studied philosophy and scholastic theology during his youth and even considered following that path before becoming a doctor (Lastres 1951a, 274). Even Unanue became interested in some theological questions, such as whether a child with two heads could also have two souls, referring to the famous case of polycephaly described by Bonet y Pueyo in his 1695 work *Desvíos de la naturaleza* (Woodham 1964, 154).

Like other enlightened intellectuals and religious figures of his time, Valdés had a deep distrust of miracles and other supernatural occurrences, whether found in the realms of popular religion or in medicine. In the case of Brother Martín de Porres, Valdés condemned the "superstitious and reprehensible credulity" of his fellow citizens, who seemed more interested in the extraordinary powers of the mulatto surgeon than in the true meaning of his actions (Valdés 1863 [1840], 120). Such credulity had figured prominently in the biographies written about him in the seventeenth century, as well as in the depositions recorded during the canonical investigation that ultimately led to his beatification. Witnesses declared that Martín de Porres occasionally levitated during prayer, was able to pass through thick walls and closed doors in order to be with those who needed his help, and could even be in several places at the same time (*Proceso* 1960, 101, 124, 147). They also stressed his subtle understanding of complex theological questions and his gift for speaking foreign languages, in spite of never having studied at a university or travelled to foreign countries (ibid., 176). He was even said to have an extraordinary ability to communicate with animals, which "searched for him and obeyed his orders as if they were endowed with reason" (ibid., 129). Despite this, it was in his role as male nurse, barber, and Romance surgeon that Martín de Porres achieved his fame as a true miracle worker. A large crowd formed each day in front of his monastery, expecting to be cured of every conceivable malady, which he reputedly achieved with his remedies, prayers, and just by laying on his hands (ibid., 124). People testified to being healed by him even after his death. On the night of his passing – a miraculous event in itself[3] – a black man named Juan Criollo recovered from a dangerous fever after having drunk a glass of water mixed with soil from the future saint's tomb (Medina 1673, 221). Later that night, a sick woman whom Martín de Porres had saved in the past was once again delivered from an illness by simply invoking him, saying, "My Father, since you are a doctor in heaven and you have restored my health on previous occasions, have mercy on me one more time" (ibid.). Many others testified to having seen Martín de Porres performing similar cures in cities far from Lima in the months following his burial (ibid., 228–9).

Valdés did not dispute that some of the cures performed by Martín de Porres were true miracles. He insisted, however, that most of them were but "the result of simple treatments whose success had to be attributed to Nature or Art" (Valdés 1863 [1840], 120). He considered only those events for which no rational explanation could be found to be "true miracles," whereas he designated those for which a natural cause, however unlikely, could be hypothesized as "apocryphal." He was of the opinion that most of the supernatural cures attributed to Martín de Porres, or to any other saint, for that matter, fell into the latter category. In this regard, Valdés's judgment did not deviate greatly from the position that the Catholic Church had mantained on miracles since the Council of Trent. Nevertheless, he did recognize a hidden risk in affirming that most of the cures performed by Martín de Porres were the result of purely natural phenomena, given their unscientific but rather effective nature; namely, he risked transforming Martín de Porres from a venerated seventeenth-century "miracle maker" into a succesful folk healer. In order to avoid the extreme of legitimizing non-scientific forms of medicine of the kind used by Dorotea Salguero, Valdés argued that Martín de Porres's use of "ineffectual remedies" was actually a façade, inspired by modesty to conceal the fact that, during prayer, God had revealed to him that his patients would recover (ibid., 125). While such a revelation of future events was certainly a supernatural gift, the actual healing of patients, as Valdés saw it, did not result from the violation of any scientific law. On the contrary, recovery was a natural process that God, in His infinite wisdom, had chosen to reveal to Martín de Porres.[4]

Miracles and cures were not the only thing that attracted Valdés to the singular mulatto surgeon. Perhaps even more importantly, he saw in Martín de Porres a figure whose religious and civic virtues could promote racial and political reconciliation and serve as a model for the republic amidst the turbulence that had followed independence.[5] With a certain degree of nostalgia, Valdés contrasted the country's bleak situation in 1839 – the year of the battle of Yungay and the end of the Bolivian-Peruvian Confederation – to the joy experienced in 1763 when, following the end of the canonical investigation, Clement XIII had declared Martín de Porres' virtues to be heroic. It was a time when, as Valdés put it, "God still looked upon Lima with pleasure" (Valdés

1863 [1840], 11). He hoped that the beatification of Martín de Porres in 1837 would work the political "miracle" of unifying all social classes behind a religious ideal and mend the many fractures caused by war and misery (ibid., 187–8). Martín de Porres's exemplary life indicated, for Valdés, as much the path towards spiritual perfection as the way towards social peace in a nation that was deeply divided along racial, economic, and ideological lines. It was also a clear indication of the potential of the *castas* to contribute to the advancement of Peru. As Manuel Antonio Urismendi put it, Martín de Porres was, despite his race, a true "Christian hero," born and raised among the poorest residents of the capital of Peru and worthy of the most sincere admiration for his patience, acceptance, and resignation, virtues that had allowed the mulatto surgeon to withstand verbal and physical abuse and create around himself an oasis of racial and social harmony (ibid., 3).

But if Valdés wrote his *Vida admirable del bienaventurado fray Martín de Porres* partly as a vindication of the religious and political role of the *castas*, it was certainly not a defence of the blacks who were still suffering from slavery. One might imagine that the issue of African slavery – still legal at the time in Peru – would figure prominently in Valdés's book, given Martín de Porres's origins and the growing international opposition to the slave trade at the time of its publication. Yet it was not so. Valdés and the Peruvian Church did not question the status quo, and in a sense they followed a path that diverged from the position of the Vatican on the issue of slavery. Gregory XVI finally made his stance clear in his encyclical *In supremo apostolatus*, written on 3 December 1839, in which he condemned all forms of slavery "as absolutely unworthy of the Christian name" and forbade "any Ecclesiastic or lay person from presuming to defend as permissible this traffic in blacks, under no matter what pretext or excuse, or from publishing or teaching in any manner whatsoever, in public or privately, opinions contrary to what We have set forth in this Apostolic Letter" (Gregory XVI 1839). Such ideas not only failed to resonate in Valdés's biography of Martín de Porres, but they were never a part of his writings or of his own personal life. In fact, Valdés had made clear his opinion about first-generation slaves in his article "Sobre las utilidades de la anatomía comprobadas con una observación" [On the usefulness of anatomy, proved with an observation] (Valdés 1792b), in which he considered them to be "for the most part of an insurmountable stupidity" (Valdés 1792b, 184).

His interest in the fate of the slave Pedro Bustamante, whom he treated for an inguineal hernia, was limited to a demonstration of what anatomy and surgery could accomplish (ibid., 184). It failed to include even a passing reference to the evils of slavery. Dávalos and Larrinaga did not actively campaign for the end of slavery either. Larrinaga's concern for Asunción, the slave woman who purportedly gave birth to a young pigeon, did not extend beyond the fact that her pregancy seemed to corroborate his own ideas on monsters and human reproduction (Larrinaga 1812). He also famously exhibited the dissected skeleton of a young slave girl, who had died just a few days after arriving in Lima, in the hospital of San Bartolomé. He did so as a way of instructing future surgeons about the complexities of human anatomy and to exemplify the fugacity of human life (Rabí Chara 2006b, 232–41). To Larrinaga's credit, however, he did at least decry the consequences of the institution of slavery in his *Apología*, in which he condemned those who thought that "one can shackle the spirit along with the hands" (Larrinaga 1791, 6). But, in general, he considered slavery more a turn of fate than a fundamental injustice and therefore he did not explicitly ask for its abolition.

Compared to Larrinaga, Valdés's position on African slavery was even more troubling. The final will and testament that he dictated to the public notary, Joaquín Luque, in 1831 demonstrates not only his acquiescence to slavery but the fact that he was a slave owner himself. As was often customary among pious slave owners, Valdés used his testament to free the slaves in his possession, but not before his death or that of his sister, whom the slaves were obliged to serve until the last days of her life. "It is my will and also that of my sister, María del Pilar Valdés," he said, "that, after her death, the two slaves that she owns and that I bought with my own money – a *moreno* named Manuel and a *zamba* named Lorenza – be freed. However, while Lorenza shall be freed immediately upon my sister's passing, Manuel should serve me until my death, after which he can also be freed. I hereby also order that all the slaves that I now own or that I might own in the future, as well as those of my sister, be freed after our passing. In order to prove their liberty, they will not be required to possess any other document beyond this one, which will be added by the notary to their acts of freedom" (Valdés 1831, 863v). Valdés later revoked this will and had two others written in the office of the public notary Gerónimo de Villafuerte (Valdés 1840, 1841). Manuel and Lorenza were not mentioned in these subsequent documents, and it is unknown whether they had died, been sold, or freed. In these later versions, Valdés did mention an old slave named Josefa Valdés who had been the property of his mother and who, on account of "her great services, faithfulness, and exemplary life" was to be given food and clothes as well as one peso each month until the day she died, without being asked to perform any services in return (Valdés 1840, 465v; 1841, 586r–v).

Valdés's actions were far from unusual among free blacks and mulattoes of comfortable economic means in Lima. Owning slaves was, at least for some of them, a sign of social prestige and a way of establishing differences among blacks, mulattoes, and *pardos* in spite of their shared African ancestry (Aguirre 1993, 292–3; Jouve Martín 2009). But they did not all decide to underline their social status by possessing slaves. In contrast to Valdés, Dávalos – who in public was silent about the issue of slavery throughout his life – left in his last will and testament a substantial amount of money as well as various properties and a well-stocked library, but no slaves (Dávalos 1821, 354r–357v; Vargas Ugarte 1943). His position was far from heroic, but the truth is that for all their admiration of José de San Martín and, later, Simón Bolívar, Valdés and Dávalos were not revolutionaries bent on abolition. As Hünefeldt has pointed out, Peru did not have a strong abolitionist movement, and when slavery was abolished in 1854, it was "almost by inertia" (Hünefeldt 1994, 3). By then, slaves had long been purchasing their freedom "with the fruits of their own labor," and an alternative workforce had become available through the importation of Chinese rural labourers (ibid., 4–5).

While Valdés's hagiography of Martín de Porres did nothing to bring about the end of slavery in Peru, his book did bring a symbolic closure to the participation of blacks and mulattoes in Peruvian medicine. Martín de Porres was the best-known black medical practitioner in early colonial Lima; Valdés was the most famous black physician in the nineteenth century. One was a humble surgeon whose miraculous cures and pious life eventually led him to sainthood; the other was a full-fledged doctor whose scientific ideas and good connections allowed him to rise to the position of *Protomédico general de la República* in one of the most turbulent periods of Peruvian history. If we are to believe the accounts of contemporary travellers and historians, in the years between Porres and Valdés there were many black and mulatto surgeons and doctors whose names and activities have mostly been lost to history. Alongside Valdés, José Manuel Dávalos and José Pastor Larrinaga became the most visible and successful representatives of that group. The three of them were, no doubt, overshadowed intellectually and politically by their white counterparts, especially by the ubiquitous figure of Hipólito Unanue. It could hardly have been otherwise in a city dominated by educated white elites and a European colonial power. But as the chapters of this book have attempted to show, Valdés, Dávalos, and Larrinaga played a fundamental role in the daily practice of medicine in colonial Lima, as well as in the reception and dissemination of the scientific revolution in Peru. Their standing in Lima's medical community allowed them to become, in turn, public writers and intellectuals.

In spite of Larrinaga's many eccentricities, his *Apología de los cirujanos del Perú* and *Cartas históricas a un amigo*, together with his efforts to create a surgical school and a charitable fund mostly for black surgeons, were singular feats at a time when most Afro-Peruvians could not read or write. Similarly, Dávalos's determination to study at Montpellier and his leading role in the smallpox vaccination campaigns of the nineteenth century speak volumes about his ability to circumvent racial legislation and navigate the complex pathways of race, identity, and scientific prestige in late-colonial Lima. The fact that Valdés was able to surpass Dávalos to become the most renowned Afro-Peruvian physician in nineteenth-century Lima is nothing less than shocking, given that Valdés began his career as a simple Latin surgeon – that is, just one step above the position held by Martín de Porres.

Despite these and other achievements, their scientific and political lives were fraught with limitations. Except for Larrinaga, they did not dare to question Unanue's hegemony over the Peruvian medical establishment; Larrinaga's fall from grace surely reminded Valdés and Dávalos of the dangers of doing so. From a political perspective, they lobbied and spoke out loudly for what they considered the constitutional rights of *pardos* and *mulatos*. Nevertheless, they quickly moved to ingratiate themselves with the most conservative sectors of colonial

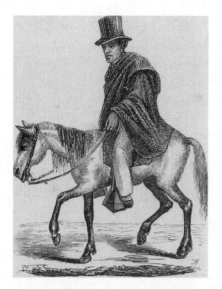 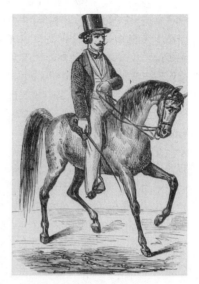

Left: "The doctor of olden times"; *right*: "The doctor of the present day."
In his book *Lima, or Sketches of the Capital of Peru,* Manuel Atanasio Fuentes
remarked that the mid-nineteenth-century doctor, in contrast to his predecessors,
distinguished himself "by the elegance of [his] garments and the beauty of his
steed; for, living at a period in which time is money, he no longer travels at
a mule's pace but at a horse's gallop" (167).

society when Ferdinand VII returned to the throne of Spain. Dávalos
and Valdés also greeted the arrival of San Martín's troops in Lima with
enthusiasm, but for all their admiration for the cause of liberty, they did
not join the liberating armies, as many black slaves did in pursuit of
freedom. Finally, while they did not renounce their racial identity, they
did everything they could to minimize it, emphasizing instead their
professional identity. These "limitations" are key to understanding how
they were able to adapt to the rapidly changing scientific and political
environment in which they lived. In fact, it was their ability to com-
promise with the established order that allowed them to negotiate their
position within the extraordinarily hierarchical world of Peruvian
medicine and to enjoy an astonishing degree of social and professional
success. Of the three, José Manuel Valdés was the most successful in
navigating these treacherous worlds of race, science, and politics.

Paradoxically, the zenith of Valdés's career, becoming Protomédico general de la República, was also the end of an era and marked the definitive expulsion of blacks and mulattoes from Peruvian medicine. Even though President Ramón Castilla declared an end to slavery on 3 December 1854, the situation for those with African ancestry did not improve, and the reality of emancipation failed to live up to the expectations generated by independence. Access to higher education continued to be restricted and remained elusive for most Afro-Peruvians. As for their role in medicine, the progress and professionalization of the medical sciences in the nineteenth century, along with the advancement of surgery, strongly contributed to the improved social standing of doctors and surgeons. As a result, the field became dominated by members of the white and *mestizo* elite, to the detriment of blacks and mulattoes, who were displaced even from the lower echelons of the medical profession. No longer did "the noble *caballeros* of Lima" look upon the profession of medicine as unworthy of them" – as something reserved mostly for blacks (Fuentes 1866a, 164). Nor was it still common to find surgeons such as Doctor Roman, "a man almost black, of middle stature, thin, with a head half covered with grey wool," making their rounds on "horses so lean that the poor beasts seemed as hollow as violins" (ibid., 165). By the mid-nineteenth century, medicine had become synonymous with social and economic success. This fact, together with the demographic decline of the Afro-Peruvian population in the first half of the century, brought an end to the era when, as Atanasio Fuentes recounted, all that was needed to become a doctor in Lima was "the inclination to do so and to be black" (Fuentes 1985 [1867], 167).

~

Notes

1 Manuel Atanasio Fuentes (1820–89) was a Peruvian doctor, university
   professor, and public intellectual well known for historical works and
   political satires in which he documented the evolution and political life
   of nineteenth-century Lima. Among his best works are *Aletazos del
   murciélago* (1866), *Lima: Apuntes históricos, descriptivos, estadísticos
   y de costumbres* (1985 [1867]), *Lecciones de jurisprudencia médica* (1875);
   and *Catecismo de Economía Política* (1877). Nevertheless, his role in the
   cultural life of Peru has been greatly overshadowed by the figure of
   Ricardo Palma, who became one of the undisputed literary figures of the
   period. For more information about Fuentes, see Núñez Hague (1998),
   Gargurevich (1999), and Herrera Cornejo (2006).

2 The text to which Archibald Smith was referring is the work of Esteban
   Terralla y Landa, who used the pseudonym Simón Ayanque to publish,
   in 1798, a collection of satirical verses entitled *Lima por dentro y por
   fuera* (Madrid: Imprenta de Villalpando). The book contains pieces of
   advice given to a hypothetical friend "who is planning to leave the City
   of Mexico and relocate in Lima." According to Terralla y Landa, in Lima
   "public health is in the hands of *negros, chinos, mulatos,* and others of
   their kind." He added that these doctors, who are "the grandsons of the
   King of Congo, are in charge of taking the pulse of little girls, ladies, and
   young men,"and he accused many of them of using false documents to
   pass as Spaniards (1798, 43, 44).

CHAPTER ONE

1 *Hermana de leche* means that they were breastfed by the same woman.
   It was common in eighteenth-century Lima to use black women, either
   enslaved or free, for the purpose of breastfeeding the offspring of wealthy
   families. As we will see in chapter 2, this practice came under attack in
   the late eighteenth century and the first decades of the nineteenth century
   when the reproduction practices of the general population came under
   the scrutiny of social and medical reformers. See Poska (2010) and Premo
   (2005a).

2 For a detailed account of Larrinaga's life, see Mendiburu (1932, 10–1)
   and Rabí Chara (2006b). Most biographical information about Larrinaga used by these two sources, including his correspondence with the
   archbishop, is provided by Larrinaga himself in his book *Cartas históricas a un amigo* (1812, 171–215). Larrinaga's self-identification as a *mulato* is clearly presented in his *Apología de los cirujanos del Perú* (1791).

3 Leaving aside notable exceptions, such as that of doctor Diego Álvarez
   Chanca, who accompanied Christopher Columbus on his second voyage
   to America, trained surgeons and physicians were not part of most ships'
   crews in the sixteenth century. It was not until 1555 that the Spanish
   Crown ordered that there be at least a barber and an apothecary onboard
   all ships involved in the *carrera de las Indias*, a regulation that affected
   only navy ships, not merchant vessels. Only in 1598 was it established
   that a physician also must be a part of their crew (Rodríguez-Sala 2011,
   6–7). Another important step was the publication in 1633 of *Ordenanzas del buen gobierno de la Armada del mar océano*, which mandated
   that all surgeons and barbers must present "letters of examination and
   approval from the doctor of the armada" in order to be allowed to practice their art (*Ordenanzas del buen gobierno* 1974 [1678], f. 30).

4 Cornelius de Pauw was not the only writer to argue in favour of the
   alleged racial and intellectual inferiority of those born in America. The
   idea that Indians and Africans were intellectually inferior to Europeans
   had appeared since the beginning of the Spanish conquest. Criticism of
   the intellectual gifts of creoles – those born in America with European
   ancestry – would become a cornerstone of the Spanish perception of the
   continent and part of the ideological justification employed by metropolitan authorities to exclude Creoles from the highest political and
   religious offices. In the eighteenth century, de Pauw's perception of an

intellectually inferior America was shared by other intellectuals of his time, particularly George Louis Leclerc, Comte de Buffon, who regarded the continent and its people as not yet having reached full maturity. For Buffon, Americans were "weaker, less active and more circumscribed in the variety of her productions" (Buffon 1791, 5: 114) than Europeans, while its indigenous people had "no vivacity, no activity of mind" (ibid., 5: 130). Guillaume Thomas François Raynal, better known as the Abbé Raynal, extended Buffon's ideas to those of European origin in his *Histoire philosophique et politique des établissements et du commerce des Européens dans les deux Indes* (1770). Echoing de Pauw, Raynal wrote that "it must be a matter of astonishment to find that America has not produced one good poet, able mathematician, nor man of genius in any single art or science" (Raynal 1777, 337).

5 According to the 1790 census, Lima had just 56 severely underpaid surgeons – the same number reported by Larrinaga in his *Apología* – and only 21 doctors to take care of the needs of a population of over 50,000 (AGI, Indiferente, 1527 [Lima, 5 December 1790]).

6 First published in 1648, Solórzano Pereyra's *Política indiana* aimed at systematizing the many laws that had been enacted for America since its discovery by Europeans. As such, it was the main existing compilation and commentary on colonial legislation until Charles II ordered the publication of *Recopilación de leyes de los Reinos de las Indias* in 1680. Book 11, Chapter xxx of Solórzano Pereyra's *Política Indiana* carried the suggestive title "Of *criollos*, *mestizos*, and *mulatos* from the Indies, about their qualities and conditions, and whether they should be considered *españoles*" (Solórzano Pereyra 1736, 1: 215). In sections 19, 20, and 21 of that chapter – the sections to which Larrinaga refers – Solórzano Pereyra considers the result of racial mixing between blacks and whites as "uglier and more extraordinary" than that of whites and Indians; but he states that "if these men were born as the result of a legitimate matrimony, and if there were not other vices or defects to be found in them, they should be considered citizens of the provinces [of the Indies] and be allowed access to the appropriate honours and offices" (ibid., 1: 217–18). In section 21, however, he warned that this was not usually the case and that *mulatos* were usually the result of "adultery and other illicit and punishable relations ... which carry with them a birth defect (*defecto de los natales*) that makes them infamous" (ibid.).

7 A *barchilón* was the person in charge of cleaning and taking care of the

basic and more physical needs of the sick. A *jeringuero* (from *jeringa*, syringe) and *untador* (from *untar*, to spread or to grease) was also a low-level medical worker, whose role was to assist nurses, surgeons, and doctors in their cures.

8 The Real Tribunal del Protomedicato was a result of the administrative reorganization undertaken by Queen Isabella of Castille and King Ferdinand of Aragon in the wake of the union of their two crowns. It was an institution whose origins lay in Aragonese laws and customs, and its modern form and structure was a result of the Royal Decree of 30 March 1477, which endowed the tribunal with the power needed to control the practice of medicine in the territories under the jurisdiction of Castille and Aragon. Protomédicos were charged with establishing the boundaries between the various medical professions. They controlled the quality of medicines sold by apothecaries, oversaw that only those with sufficient knowledge were certified, and ensured that only those of appropriate racial, religious, and familial lineage could practise medicine. The definitive reorganization of the Tribunal del Protomedicato, which survived, with minor changes, until the end of the colonial period, took place under Phillip II in 1588. For more information, see Campos Díez (1996, 43–58), Lanning (1985, 14–23), and Riera Palmero (2000).

9 To the dismay of its many advocates, the progress of academic medicine in Peru was sluggish during the sixteenth century and the first decades of the seventeenth century. The first attempts to establish a chair of medicine date from 1568, when the licentiate Lope García de Castro – who became governor of Peru upon the death of Viceroy Conde de Nieva in 1564 – asked Phillip II to install the chair at San Marcos (Delgado Matallana and Rabí Chara 2006, 17). Although his request was granted, it was not until 1576, when Antonio Sánchez de Renedo – who had arrived in 1569 to become protomédico – began to teach *Prima de Medicina* (princioales of medicine). Renedo's designation was far from surprising, given the growing interest of the Spanish Crown in American medicinal plants and their use. In 1570 Phillip II had included among the tasks given to protomédicos a mandate to learn about and take deposition of "all Spanish and Indian doctors, surgeons, herbalists, and other persons of interest who might know something about the medicinal herbs, trees, plants, and seeds that are in the province of their jurisdiction. Also, they will inform themselves about the experience of those things, how they are used and the quantities in which they are adminis-

tered, how they are cultivated, and whether they grow in dry or humid places" (*Recopilación de leyes de los Reinos de las Indias*, libro v, título vi, Ley i). Sánchez de Renedo's tenure as chair of Prima de Medicina was unfortunately short. After his death in 1578, the position was occupied only intermittently owing to lack of funding. This bleak scene appears not to have affected the Spanish metropolitan authorities, since it was not until 1634 that Viceroy Count of Chinchón formally established the chair of Prima de Medicina and designated his personal doctor, Juan de la Vega, for the job. De la Vega's position was followed that same year by the creation of a professorship in *Vísperas de Medicina* (Vespers) which was bestowed upon doctor Jerónimo Andrés Rocha. A request for the creation of a chair of Método de Galeno – to be devoted to the study of the works of Hippocrates, Galen, Avicenna, and Mercado, among others – was sent to Spain in 1660, but not until 1690 did the professorship become a reality, with the appointment of Dr Francisco Vargas Machuca (Lastres 1951a, 130). The creation of a chair in Anatomy took even longer. Despite having been requested in 1660, along with the chair of Método de Galeno, it was not formally established until 1711. Furthermore, those who believed that anatomy would at last be taught in Peru after such a long wait were in for a disappointment. The position was not filled until 1723, and even then anatomy was only irregularly taught until 1752, when sufficient funds were allocated to endow the chair (ibid., 193).

10 The fact that hospitals were a racial "melting pot" does not mean that racial, social, and economic hierarchies were not observed. Health professionals were remunerated according to their rank. In the Hospital Real de San Andrés, a doctor was paid 600 pesos, a surgeon, 400 (the same as an apothecary), a male nurse, 200, and a barber even less: 150 (Cobo 1882 [1639], 306). For a discussion of the evolution of these and other hospitals in colonial Lima, see Lastres 1951a, 39–49; Cahill 1995, 123–54; and Rabi Chara 2006a, 173–83.

11 First- and second-generation black slaves retained part of their African ethnic identity. Black brotherhoods "painted the walls of their meeting-houses with scenes evoking their African past and at their Sunday meetings, after discussing brotherhood business, they sang and danced into the evening to the music of African instruments. At public festivals they paraded as 'nations' (ethnic groups) wearing African dress, playing African music, and performing African war-dances" (Higgins 2010, 77).

Ethnic identities tended to disappear after the second generation. In the case of individuals of mixed Spanish and African descent, such as *mulatos,* identity was based on *casta* more than on the ethnic origins of their ancestors. If anything, they frequently chose to highlight their European rather than African roots (see Jouve Martín 2007, 179–201).

12 It was only in 1606 when a formal brotherhood was set up. The new administration took steps to improve the building and moved the rooms for the sick away from the church to an area better ventilated (Warren 2004, 49–50).

13 As van Deusen remarked, the founders of the hospital "did not exaggerate when they stressed that people went there to die. Nearly thirty percent of the free persons of colour (396 of 1,333) and one-quarter of all slaves (202 of 859) never left the hospital. Of these, forty percent survived less than a week, and most were dead within a month" (van Deusen 1991, 27). Bleak as these statistics were, they represented an improvement on the previous situation of most freed slaves.

14 Information about the life of Brother Martín de Porres comes from the seventeenth-century biography *Vida prodigiosa del venerable siervo de Dios fr. Martín de Porres* (1673) by Bernardo de Medina, as well as the extensive documentation compiled for Martín de Porras's beatification process (see *Proceso de beatificación de fray Martín de Porras* 1960). Busto Durthurburu (2006) draws extensively from these two sources.

15 Unsurprisingly, Latin surgeons viewed the far less prepared Romance surgeons and bloodletters with contempt. This contempt was echoed in the mid-nineteenth century by Atanasio Fuentes, who did not hesitate to point out that a Romance surgeon "was received after a few months' practice at the hospital, and provided he was able to distinguish the cases in which a poultice of marsh-mallows was preferable to one of bread and milk, he was sure to obtain his diploma from the worthy *Tribunal del Protomedicato*" (Fuentes 1866a, 164).

16 The census bore the title *Plan demostrativo de la población comprehendida en el recinto de la ciudad de Lima, con distinción de clases y estados, instruido sobre datos de la enumeración total de sus individuos* [Illustrative plan of the comprehensive population in the precincts of the city of Lima, according to class and state distinctions, appraised using data on the total number of its inhabitants] (AGI, Indiferente, 1527 [Lima, 5 December 1790]). It was submitted to the Spanish Crown along with a commentary on the results that apppeared in the *Mercurio peru-*

ano on 3 February 1791 entitled "Reflexiones históricas y políticas sobre el estado de la población de esta capital" [Historical and political reflections on the state of this capital's population]. Despite the claims of accuracy, the authors acknowledged that "it is not unknown to us that some neighbours, be it because of chance or malice, did not report to the census takers the complete number of individuals [under their care,] especially slaves; but we do not believe that more than 2,000 people could have been hidden from us" ("Reflexiones históricas y políticas" 1791, 93-4). The census contained several arithmetic errors and inaccuracies, (for a discussion of those inaccuracies see Pérez Cantó 1982, 385; Anna 1975, 234-5). Nevertheless, the final document provides us with a relatively precise description of race in late colonial Lima.

17 Biographical data about José Manuel Valdés come from different sources. Some of the most important are the testaments that he dictated a few years before his death (Valdés 1831, 1840, 1841). As was relatively common in the case of mestizos and mulattoes of high social standing, these documents do not refer to Valdés's race. He does, however, refer to himself as a mulatto in some of his writings, particularly in his *Vida admirable del bienaventurado fray Martín de Porras* (1863, 9). He was widely identified as a mulatto by his contemporaries and later biographers. One particularly important biographer is José A. Lavalle, who wrote a small work in 1863 entitled *El doctor don José Manuel Valdés: Apuntes sobre su vida y sus obras*. He expanded the information contained in this text some time later in a work of the same title (Lavalle n.d.). For more information about Valdés, see Lastres 1951b; 129-46; Mendiburu 1890, 8:219-22; Romero 1942, 296-319; and López Martínez 1993.

18 Other than the individuals whom Valdés references in his writings, it is difficult to establish exactly who was part of his clientele. Apart from the testimony of his contemporaries, who attest to the high esteem in which he was held by Lima's upper class, most information comes from the cases that Valdés himself refers to in his writings. An exception to this is found in AGN (CA-JO 1, 137, 2490, 1798, f. 1), in which a certain Agustín de la Fuente asks Valdés to testify about his illness and states that he had been under his care.

19 For the study of the life and academic career of Dávalos, see Mendiburu 1878, 3: 1; Lastres 1951a, 265-8; and Vargas Ugarte 1943, 325-42. For his testament, see Dávalos 1821.

20 The competition for this chair illustrates how rapidly social relations could change in colonial Lima. Dávalos argued during his defence that the position should not be given to "don Juan Tafalla, since he had devoted his career entirely to the army and not to the study of Botany, and the King had only ordered him to be a favoured candidate if there were no other party more qualified for the post" (quoted in F. Herrera 1937, 56). In the end, Tafalla was awarded the position "as a reward for the services he rendered during the Ruiz y Pavón scientific expedition, in their long pilgrimages through our national territory" (ibid.).

21 The renewal of the medical and physical sciences started under the patronage of the last Habsburg king, Charles II (Cañizares Esguerra 2006, 46–63; De Vos 2006, 61). The Crown's "early, active, and abiding interest in natural resources and medicine" (De Vos 2006, 60) led it to sponsor major scientific expeditions to Peru, such as those led by La Condamine and Jorge Juan de Ulloa, and later by those of other Enlightenment travellers such as Alexander von Humboldt. Early efforts reached "their greatest maturity and mobilization, however, only during the reign of Charles III, especially after the *comercio libre* decree of 1778" (ibid., 64). Medicine was of particular interest during these expeditions, and shipments of American herbal medicines were regularly sent to Spain from the 1740s onwards (ibid.).

22 Bueno combined Sydenham's eclecticism with Boerhaave's and de Haen's emphasis on clinical demonstrations. Sydenham had argued that a doctor's place was at the side of the sick. As he put it to the young Hans Sloane, "You must go to the bedside, it is there alone you can learn disease" (quoted in Cunningham 1989, 183). This advice might seem obvious today, but as Cunnigham has pointed out, for most seventeenth- and eighteenth-century physicians, the curing of an illness depended on the physicians understanding "*how the human body works*, and how *drugs work* in the human body," and as a result "there was neither room nor occasion for *experimenta*; nor was there any particular need for *new* observations; and given the large numbers of practical medical books with authoritative guidance in them that one could consult, there was specially no need for *one's own* observations! The *theory* one had been brought up on told one all one needed to know" (ibid., 177). Sydenham did not advocate a particular system to remedy this situation. On the contrary, he adopted an eminently practical approach. For him, "an experiment at the bedside consisted of nothing more sophisticated than

trial and error in the administration of drugs and of medical techniques such as bleeding or purging. If a treatment seemed to be working, it was continued with, if not it was dropped" (ibid., 186). Boerhaave had made the clinic "the basis for the curriculum" and taught students to judge "each case individually and follow carefully all changes in the patient's condition as medications were applied" (Burke 1977, 32). Boerhaave's *Institutiones medicae* (1708) – a synthesis of contemporary knowledge on anatomy, physiology, and chemistry that offered a classificatory system of disease – and his *Aphorisms* (1709), a practical guide with clinical advice, became very popular in Peru and Mexico, as well as in other parts of the Spanish empire until the nineteenth century.

23 Established in 1711, the chair in Anatomy at San Marcos only became functional by the mid-eighteenth century. The construction of an anatomical amphitheatre was postponed until the 1790s, and an independent school of medicine and surgery did not exist until the 1810s. This situation contrasts with the influence of the Vesalian movement in Spain in the sixteenth century (López Piñero 1979, 45). In Lima, the main problem was not academic in nature (Vesalius's teachings were known through the works of Spanish commentators); rather, it was financial. A lack of funds, not lack of interest, prevented the systematic teaching and research of anatomy in Peru (Dávila Condemarín 1854, 5–27; Valdizán 1927, 1: 17–156). The publication in Lima of Federico Bottoni's *Evidencia de la circulación de la sangre* in 1723 helped to disseminate Harvey's theories on blood circulation as an undoubted scientific truth, giving further impetus to the study of anatomy in the viceroyalty. Bottoni's work led Juan de Avedaño y Campoverde, chair of Vísperas de Medicina at San Marcos, to conclude that "while medicine has evolved over the centuries, anatomy seems to have reached its perfection only in our age" (Bottoni 1723, iv). By the second half of the eighteenth century, books like those by Martín Martinez, *Anatomía completa del hombre* (1728), and Jacques-Benigne Winslow, *Exposition anatomique de la structure du corps humain* (1732), had become common reference texts in the education of Peruvian physicians. Dr Francisco Matute taught anatomy at San Marcos in the 1770s through the use of cadavers and had "the distinction, and no doubt pleasure, of seeing his colleagues, whose scholastic conceptions made them admirers of prestige, accept his word with the same credulity which had made them defer formerly to the scholastic authorities" (Lanning 1940, 107). Even the church showed an

increased awareness of the relevance of anatomy and surgery, exemplified by the friar Francisco González Laguna's 1781 publication of a medical-theological treatise on caesarian sections entitled *El zelo sacerdotal para con los niños no-nacidos* (priestly zeal for the unborn children).

1 There were many who shared Unanue's belief that surgery had been known in the viceroyalty "only by name" before the eighteenth century (Unanue 1793a, 106–7; Haenke 1901, 83). To a certain extent, Unanue's dismissal of pre-1700 surgery in Peru was unjustified. It is true that seventeenth-century surgeons lacked a coherent *modus operandi* and that many in Lima practised their art without proper training, but that does not mean that the city's surgeons lacked public recognition. One renowned *limeño* surgeon was Pedro Gago de Vadillo. In 1630 he published his *Luz de la verdadera cirugía*, a comprehensive volume on the nature of wounds and their remedies, which remained highly influential in the Spanish empire throughout the colonial period. His treatise relied heavily on the *Thesoro de la verdadera cirugía* (1604), a work by the Sevillian surgeon Bartolomé Hidalgo de Agüero, who was known as the *Pareo español*, or Spanish Paré (Gómez Ocaña 1912, 90).

2 The renown of French surgery was in no small part cemented by the fame of Charles François Félix, who in 1686 had successfully operated on Louis XIV of France for an anal fistula, after having practised the procedure on several peasants. This helped make Félix a wealthy man and a member of the nobility. It also contributed to the prestige of surgery in France, culminating in the creation of the Académie royale de chirurgie in 1731 under the direction of the royal surgeons Georges Mareschal (1658–1736) and François Gigot de la Peyronie (1678–1747). The prestige of French doctors further manifested itself in the pages of the *Mercurio peruano*. According to Clement, French doctors were the most commonly cited authors by nationality (with 18.3% of the total), followed by Peruvians (14.6%), and Italians (14.2%) (Clement 1997, 122).

3 Valdés's first articles for the *Mercurio*, which appeared on 5 June and 25 December 1791, dealt with the reform and regulation of childbirth. Tellingly, the first part of his observations appeared under the heading of "hygiene." Valdés's third article, which was published on 2 February 1792, was devoted to an entirely different topic: animal venoms and their

remedies. His fourth "letter" (19 July 1792) dealt with the usefulness of anatomy, while the fifth and sixth (10 and 13 October 1793) were written in response to a question raised during one of his demonstrations at the anatomical amphitheatre concerning the use of "fixed air," or carbon dioxide, in the treatment of dysentery.

Larrinaga submitted a surgical dissertation about an abnormal birth entitled "Surgical dissertation on a nine-month-old fetus born to a woman through her urethra," which was published in three parts (31 May, 3 June, and 7 June 1792). This article was followed several months later (9 and 12 August 1792) by letters discussing whether a woman could be transformed into a man. Larrinaga also published a brief surgical dissertation on aneurisms on 22 November 1792 and 12 May 1793, and submitted a defence of his scientific observations against the harsh criticism that they had received in an anonymous letter submitted to the *Mercurio* the previous February. In their texts, Larrinaga and Valdés saw it as their obligation to put their knowledge of the latest medical theories and surgical techniques at the service of the general population rather than engaging in specialized forms of scientific writing. The two mulatto surgeons found an intellectual role model for their work in Hipólito Unanue, who "never considered himself exclusively a physician, and indeed, rarely spoke of himself as such, usually preferring the label 'philosopher,' or more modestly, 'writer'" (Woodham 1970, 694). As if attempting to prove that he was not only a gifted surgeon but also an accomplished humanist, Larrinaga published a historical poem that focused on the history of the Incas in Peru and appeared on 9 September 1792, followed by another poetic composition (7 March 1792) focusing on the Spanish viceroys who had governed Peru.

4 Most articles dealing with medicine were published by Unanue, either under his real name (6) or under his pseudonym Aristio (8). The number by Valdés (5) and Larrinaga (4) were followed by Hesperófilo [José Rossi y Rubí] (4), Nolasco Crespo (3), Hermágoras [José L. Egaña] (2), and Philaletes (2). Other contributors were Pinacio Montano (1), Ignacio Castro (1), Joseph Coquette (1), Felipe Llanos (1), Pedro Fernández (1), Celestino Mutis (1), Meligario (1), Thimeo (1), Teagnes (1), Chiros-atychio Prebyographo (1), and Francisco Rebollar (1). A total of ten articles were published anonymously (see Clement 1979, 79–81). The medical topics addressed in the journal included the development of anatomy, the inauguration of the anatomical amphitheatre, altitude sickness, old

age and longevity, an extraordinary case of colic, a case of solitaria, an aneurism of the lower lip, dysentery, thermal waters, animal venom, the treatment of diverse illnesses from surrounding regions, the properties of quinine, or cinchona bark, mineral waters, the virtues of the coca plant, the variety of patients at Lima's hospitals, hygienic methods for the maintenance of good health for pregnancies, and other medical curiosities (Pamo Reyna 2000, 1341–2).

5 The regulations of the Sociedad académica de Amantes del País made it almost impossible for two mulatto surgeons to become part of it, no matter how well prepared they were from an intellectual point of view. According to the regulations, the society consisted of a president, a vice-president, two censors, two secretaries, a treasurer, a press secretary and three different kinds of member: academic fellows, consulting fellows, and honourary fellows (Cerdán y Pontero 1794, 138). The number of academic fellows, all experts in their fields, was limited to thirty, at least twenty-one of whom were required to have their residence in Lima. The number of consulting fellows was limited to sixteen well-prepared individuals, who had the task of helping the intellectual work of their academic peers. In order to become either an academic or a consulting fellow, a nominee needed to obtain both a majority vote in the society's assembly and the approval of the viceroy. Finally, honourary members were named by a majority vote at the society's discretion. Even if the regulations did not exclude those of mixed European and African descent, the kind of support necessary to become a member, and the veto power of the viceroy, made it highly unlikely that a non-white would be accepted. It is therefore not surprising that the names of José Pastor Larrinaga and José Manuel Valdés do not appear among the society's fellows (*Sociedad académica de Amantes del País* 1793, 19–24).

6 Larrinaga was referring to Diego de Velasco and Francisco Villaverde's *Curso teórico práctico de cirujía en que se contienen los más célebres descubrimientos modernos* [Surgical course of theory and praxis containing the most celebrated modern discoveries] (1763), a reference work written in late-eighteenth-century Spain by two surgery professors from the Reales colegios de cirugía de Barcelona and Cádiz, respectively. For a discussion of the technique used by Larrinaga, see Velasco and Villaverde (1763, 489–97).

7 Joseph Black, who studied many of its properties, coined the term "fixed air" although it was also known as "wild spirit" (*spiritus sylvestre*) by

van Helmont, "mefitic acid" by Morveau, "mefitic gas" by Macquez, "aerial acid" by Bergman, and "carbonic acid" by Fourcroy (Valdés 1793, 94). Following Lavoisier, Valdés estimated the concentration of "fixed air" in the atmosphere at 1%, with vital air (27%) and *azote* [nitrogen] (72%) comprising the remainder (Valdés 1793, 94).

8 According to Unanue, the corpse in question belonged to a European male about forty years old, who had suffered from dysentery for about three months and had been treated in the Hospital de San Andrés. In the postmortem, the internal organs such as the liver, pancreas, and kidneys were found to be in good condition, but the intestines were severely affected by gangrene. The gangrene was particularly noticeable in the colon, the cecum, and the rectum, while the gastrointestinal tract was completely reduced to putrid mucus (Unanue 1793b, 129–30). Unanue believed that his observations confirmed Pringle and Cullen's theories, wherein "the large intestines [constituted] the principal site of dysentery" and "the rectum and lower part of the colon are the most exposed to gangrene" (ibid.). Unanue complemented his observations with a second article "Indagaciones sobre la disentería y el vicho. Observación 2da exraida de las que se han hecho en el Real anfiteatro anatómico" entitled [Investigations on dysentery and 'vicho.' Secondary observations taken from the Royal Anatomical Amphitheatre] (Unanue 1793c).

9 Commonly found on the warm and humid plains of the Orinoco and Amazon river basins, the *enfermedad del vicho* was a malignant fever that was similar to dysentery in that it caused a distension of the anal sphincter along with rectal gangrene. Described by Joseph Gumilla in his *Historia natural, civil y geográfica de las naciones situadas en las riveras del río Orinoco* [Natural, civil and geographic history of the nations situated on the tributaries of the Orinoco River] (1791), the *enfermedad del vicho* was a malady common to the tropical forests of the Amazon and Orinico rivers. The general population, along with most educated people, believed that it was caused by "a small living animal, born in the intestines, or living there invasively," hence the name *vicho* (meaning an insect). Gumilla, however, considered the malady a kind of tropical fever. Its symptoms were "a high fever, accompanied by exhaustion and sleepiness so deep that it is impossible for the patients to wake up or even open their eyes; at the same time the patients' hemorrhoidal muscles become greatly relaxed and there is a laxative effect; the laxative process can be fomented with repeated administrations of lemon

slices, and if the patient is made to swallow this bitter fruit, he will soon recover; but if the remedy is not given quickly, twelve hours after the first complaint the patient's left arm will begin to tremble; afterwards there will be a minor trembling in the right arm; later the patient's thumbs will begin to tremble and curl; and finally all the fingers will be curled tightly against the patient's palms; after twenty-four hours patients will certainly die, preceded by strong convulsions in every limb of their body" (Gumilla 1791, 202–3).

The remedies used to cure the *enfermedad del vicho*, along with their use for the treatment of dysentery, were widely criticized by Unanue, Valdés, and many other Lima physicians (Unanue 1790b, 130; "Resultado" 1791, 128). In most cases, the recommendations made by physicians were disregarded, and the ignorance of the populace drove them to prefer the advice of charlatans to that of doctors. The harm caused by the public's failure to recognize the appropriate treatments for dysentery and the *enfermedad del vicho* was significant. As Philaletes lamented, "Dear God! What effect will frequent doses of putrid urine, olive broth, astringent concoctions with Egyptian ointment, turpentine, spirits, gunpowder, lemon, and other similar drugs have on inflamed intestines! ... We must completely open the people's eyes: there is no such Vicho amongst us. This illness does not exist in our Court: the dysentery that afflicts us requires a method of treatment that is completely contrary, and only the enlightened Professor knows the required administration" (Philaletes 1793a, 145–6).

10 Unanue and Valdés did not completely rule out the use of popular remedies for this kind of malady; in fact, they praised some of them. Unanue particularly favoured what he called an "excellent practice," which required the administration of certain remedies used by "many people in the surrounding villages and estates" and involved providing patients in the early stages of dysentery with "large repeated doses of almond oil, because this relaxes the intestines, expels fecal material, and protects the stomach lining from the first effects of the stimulant that can cause their putrefaction" (Unanue 1793b, 130).

11 An alternative and increasingly popular way of treating dysentery was with a preparation that contained mercury. A description of the method – which was strongly rejected by Valdés later in his career – appeared in the *Mercurio peruano* on 17 October 1793 in an article entitled "New Method to Cure Dysentery." The author, who submitted the text anony-

mously, claimed that the method had been explained to him by Pedro María González, a surgeon in the Royal Spanish Navy (one of the overseas surgeons so despised by Larrinaga), who in turn had learned it from English physicians working in New Spain. According to the article, mercury could be administered as a saline preparation in pill form, as long as "the stomach conserved enough energy and elasticity to digest them," or through ointments applied to "the site where the pains are most active and lasting" ("Resultado" 1791, 105)

12 It could hardly have been otherwise, since it took the scientific establishment in Spanish America some time to realize the full extent of Lavoisier's theories. Although an article published in 1792 in the *Mercurio peruano* summarized some of his main ideas, his book *Traité élémentaire de la chimie* (1789) was not published in Spanish translation until 1797 (Bifano & Whittembury 2007, 281).

13 According to Fragoso, men "do not differ from women apart from the fact that their genitals are outside their bodies. If we were to perform an anatomical investigation of a maiden, we would find that she has two testicles, two seminal vesicles, and an organ of the same shape as a man's penis. Therefore, if, after having produced a perfect man, Nature wished to transform him into a woman, it would suffice to insert her genitals back inside her body. And, conversely, if it wished to transform her back into a man, all Nature would have to do is pull the genitals back out" (Fragoso 1627 [1586], 162).

14 Larrinaga's reasoning reflected the increasing medical and philosophical attention devoted to female genitalia, especially the clitoris, ever since the sixteenth century when Gabriel Fallopius and Renauldus Columbus produced the first modern descriptions of the organ. Their "discoveries" spurred a renewed interest in the "abnormalities" and "monstrosities" associated with female genitalia.

15 According to Larrinaga, this was a condition that was particularly common in Africa, where doctors loudly announced their presence in the streets "so that those unfortunate women suffering under the weight and magnitude of such excrescencies could hear the comforting call of those who, armed with a knife, were ready to relieve their suffering" (Larrinaga 1792b, 235–6).

16 The writer, lexicographer, and chaplain to King Phillip II, Sebastián de Covarrubias, published in his widely circulated work *Emblemas morales* (1610) an emblem that depicted the confusion that such deviations from

Nature created, and he accompanied it with the following legend: "I am a *hic*, and *haec*, and *hoc*. / I confess I am a man, I am a woman, I am a third, / Who is neither the one nor the other, and it is not clear / Which of these things he is. I am a terror / For those who believe me to be a horrendous and rare monster" (Covarrubias 1610, 164; translation by Horswell 2005, 63).

17 Larrinaga's enumeration serves as a good guide to the authors who influenced educated surgeons in late-eighteenth-century Lima. According to him, the only case that resembled the one he described was found in Juan de Dios López's *Compendio anatómico* (1785,176), which cited a report by Alexis Littré about a 32-year-old woman who "expelled the bones of a six-month-old fetus through her anus" (Larrinaga 1792a, 73–4; Dios López 1785, 167–9). For a contemporary take on the issue, see Atug et al. (2005).

18 Aristotle's complete quotation is "Natura daemonia est, non divina." It comes from *De divinatione per somnum* (Aristotle 1831, 239). History offered several examples of nature breaking its own rules. Larrinaga himself mentioned, among others, the case of Catalina de Medicis, wife of Henry II, who was unable to conceive during the first ten years of her marriage but then became so fertile that "she gave birth to five princes and five princesses." He also referred to the case described by Pierre Dionos of a woman in Tolosa (Spain) who discovered that she had carried a fetus in her abdomen for twenty-five years which was born half petrified and weighed eight pounds. Larrinaga also mentioned Phillip Salmuthi, who claimed in his *Observationum medicarum centuriae tres posthumæ* (1648) to have witnessed an abortion "through the mouth and through the anus," respectively (Larrinaga 1792a, 66–8).

19 The Crown was in full agreement. Improving the health and birth rate of children, particularly "Spanish" children, was already part of imperial policy (Premo 2005b). As González has noted, the control of reproduction became part "of the very process of creating an empire, of establishing the cultural and social boundaries of life in the Indies, as well as the racial and political domination of Europeans over others" (González 2007, 7).

20 As a general rule, Valdés claimed that women should be bled before the third month of pregnancy, as should those who continued to menstruate in spite of their pregnancy. A pregnant woman should also be bled "every time she evinces a surplus of blood, which manifests itself in the form of

headaches, lack of sleep, difficulty breathing, hot flashes, a very strong pulse, etc." (Valdés 1791a, 95). Valdés warned, however, that without these symptoms bloodletting was useless and could be harmful unless the patient suffered from an illness that required it.

21 Midwives were not the only "plague" affecting Peruvians in the eyes of the editors of the *Mercurio*. Even if Valdés opted not to comment on the subject, the debate concerning midwives was closely related to another colonial controversy: the use of black and *mulata* women as wet nurses for Spanish children. Considered widely prevalent and extremely undesirable, wet nurses were viewed as a means "through which slaves and free blacks and *castas* could exercise their pernicious influence" (Warren 2004, 83). By the end of the eighteenth century, the issue had become "a lightning rod for political commentary about the racial order of late colonial society," and local papers began "to focus on the intimacy forged between colonial servants and creole children and published articles in which authors wondered if wet nursing in particular had become a degenerative force that corrupted and stunted the colonies" (Premo 2005a, 243).

22 Levret was particularly well known for his designs of obstetric instruments, but this was a topic that Valdés may have considered too specialized for the readership of the *Mercurio peruano* (Valdés 1791b, 194). He also made reference to another famous French surgeon, Julien Clement, who was widely known for helping deliver the illegitimate son of Madame de La Vallière and Louis XIV in 1663 (Bancroft-Livingston 1956, 261–7).

23 Many conditions could prevent normal cervical dilation and lead to a miscarriage. Among them, Valdés singled out the excess of blood in the uterine vessels and the obstruction of the intestines or the bladder; he provided advice on how to treat these problems and detailed the conditions under which bloodletting should be performed to facilitate birth (Valdés 1791b, 194).

24 Estimates of the amount of blood in the human body were not the only calculations that Philaletes criticized in his article. Larrinaga had argued that, since the heart filled with 4 Castillian ounces of blood per diastole (beat), it was able to circulate all of the body's blood, or 128 Castillian ounces, after just 32 diastoles (1 Castillian pound = 16 Castillian ounces). Following James Keill's estimates of the normal rate of heart beats per minute, Larrinaga had claimed that the heart was able to move as much

as 80 Castillian ounces of blood in just half a minute and potentially more than that in the case of abnormally high pulses, such as those of patients with fevers (Larrinaga 1792d, 207). For Philaletes, even if one was to concede that there were no more than 128 ounces (8 pounds) of blood in the human body, Larrinaga had still grossly neglected the fact that the velocity at which blood passes through the heart depends on its location in the body: "Each body part has its own particular circuit, and not all are of equal velocity, with higher speeds in the areas closer to the heart, and much slower velocities in the more distant parts, flowing easily in the lungs and the brain, and more slowly in the liver and glands, (and) extremely slow in the bones" (Philaletes 1793a,141).

25 Drawing on his research with animals, Almeida established that the blood present in a human body was around "a twentieth part of its total weight: such that people commonly weighing 140 to 160 pounds will have about 8 pounds or 128 ounces of blood maximum" (Larrinaga 1793b, 31). Regarding the amount of blood that enters the heart with each diastole, Almeida referred to his experiments with dogs, in which he had introduced a blood coagulant through their jugular arteries. When the liquid reached the hearts' ventricles, it "coagulated the blood it found there, which being coagulated could not exit through the pulmonary artery." After dissecting the dogs to examine their hearts, he found six ounces of blood in their right ventricles, sometimes even more. After accounting for the larger size of a human heart and the fact that the dog's heart had swollen as a result of the procedure, Larrinaga concluded that it was prudent to estimate that "there would be at least four ounces of blood in the heart's right ventricle with each diastole" (Larrinaga 1793b, 32; Almeida 1792, 273).

26 Even when it did not advocate radical political change, the reformist ideals that had sustained the *Mercurio peruano* – freedom of speech and the creation of an enlightened, merit-based society – were ultimately at odds with the more traditional beliefs of Lima's aristocracy, as was its exaltation of Peruvian identity, which has frequently been cited as an example of the emergence of a creole protonational consciousness and a forerunner of the political thought that eventually led to independence (Belaunde 1987, 239).

27 This was especially true of José Manuel Valdés, who eventually, in 1794, was invited by Unanue to participate in a series of clinical lectures at the anatomical amphitheatre, a "grand project that was proposed many

times and also abandoned many times owing to the difficulty of the endeavour" (Unanue 1794, 195–6). A sign of Larrinaga's fall from grace with Unanue after his controversy with Philaletes is that Unanue invited José Manuel Dávalos to join Valdés in the anatomical lectures instead of him, even though Dávalos had not contributed a single piece to the *Mercurio peruano*.

CHAPTER THREE

1 Brother Matías del Carmen Verdugo, a doctor educated in Chile, seems to have been the first physician to administer smallpox inoculations in the Spanish colonies. In the 1770's Domingo de Soria suggested carrying out inoculations in Lima, and Cosme Bueno printed a formal opinion addressing the issue (Lanning 1940, 120–1). As for Belomo, the fact that he was a peninsular Spaniard and a surgeon did not prevent him from becoming a successful member of Lima's medical elite. As Warren points out, doctors in Lima spoke of Belomo "as one of their own, praised his knowledge of medicine, and eventually appointed him to the position of surgeon examiner (*protocirujano*)" (Warren 2010, 79).

2 Valdés based his medical opinions on his own observations as well as on Jean Astruc's *Tractatus de morbis mulierum* (1763) and William Rowley's *The Rational Practice of Physic* (1793). Valdés found Astruc's treatise useful as a theoretical framework, but he faulted him for "not having seen or cured" uterine cancer. Rowley's doctrines, on the contrary, were empirical and "based on observations," but the English physician dealt only with varieties of uterine cancer that were infrequently observed among the women of Lima (Valdés 1815c, 100; Rowley 1793, 1: 442). The treatises of Astruc and Rowley were more valuable as texts that disseminated medical knowledge rather than as breakthrough scientific contributions. A renowned physician with a long list of publications, Jean Astruc was better known to posterity for his theological writings on the Book of Genesis than for his medical opinions. For his part, William Rowley, "a man of no high reputation, but of a very active pen, writing medical treatises for popular reading" (Fox 1901, 54), became known for a series of controversies with the Scottish anatomist and physician William Hunter, the leading obstetrician of his day. In addition to *The Rational Practice of Physic* (1793), Rowley penned a work about the diseases specific to women entitled *A Treatise*

on *Female, Nervous, Hysterical, Hypochondriacal, Bilious, Convulsive Diseases; Aoplexy and Palsy; with Thoughts on Madness, Suicide, etc.* (1788). Like his observations on the effects of the copaiba balsam, Valdés's treatise on uterine cancer was published only in 1815 as part of his *Disertaciones médico-quirúrgicas* (1815c).

3 Based on Unanue's interest in recruiting students from other regions of the viceroyalty and his tolerant attitude towards students from other racial groups, historians such as Rodriguez Merino have controversially proposed that Unanue originally envisioned the Colegio de medicina y cirugía de San Fernando as actively pursuing racial integration and political emancipation. According to Rodríguez Merino, Unanue's desire to extend modern science to every corner of Peru was accompanied by the hidden goal of "liberating the Peruvian people from the discrimination and servitude under which they lived" and putting into practice "the principles of liberty, equality, and fraternity proclaimed by the declaration of the Rights of Man and the French Revolution" (Rodríguez Merino 1990, 532).

4 While Unanue's proposal was indeed progressive, it did not signal the Copernican change to Peruvian medicine and science he had expected. The project was heavily influenced by the work of Herman Boerhaave and the Leiden School, whose theories were at least fifty years old by that time (Pamo Reina 2009, 64; Lanning 1940, 109). Even worse, much of the curriculum never went beyond the planning stages because of a lack of funds and lack of faculty members suitaably trained to teach the proposed subjects (ibid.). The Junta superior de medicina y cirugía de Cádiz considered Unanue's proposal too ambitious, more suitable for a university than for a relatively small medical school. It also raised doubts about the appropriateness of the curriculum and expressed concern that the large number of subjects would prevent students from obtaining the set of skills needed to become successful physicians (Warren 2010, 208–10). According to Warren, Unanue and the rest of the faculty of the future Colegio de medicina y cirugía de San Fernando dismissed most of the recommendations of the Junta superior "out of both local pride and the desire, as creole doctors, to defend their medical and scientific expertise as equal or superior to that of doctors in Spain. Having for years declared themselves the patriotic champions of enlightened local and regional science in the colony, they interpreted the *junta*'s suggestions as an affront to their authority and an act of condescension" (ibid.).

5 The salary of doctors and surgeons was usually established in hospital constitutions, but Larrinaga also gives us an idea of how much a surgeon earned at the end of the eighteenth century. According to him, the salary paid to a surgeon who worked in a hospital was "barely eight to ten pesos a month. There were, he said "many young individuals who work as surgeons not because of this poor salary, but for the satisfaction of being useful to their homeland, their parents, and their acquaintances" (1791, 30).

6 Such was the case with the article "Descripción anatómica de un monstruo," published on 2 January 1791, in which the author – who used the pseudonym "Thimeo" – described the birth of an "extremely frightening" child to a black slave named Mariana. The child had no brain, lacked a forehead and other parts of the skull, was missing several key organs, and had two sets of genitalia, but was inexplicably born alive (Thimeo 1791, 8; Meléndez 2011, 138). On 18 March 1792, Unanue himself published a reflection on monsters. Entitled "Descripción de un ternero bicipite seguida de algunas reflexiones sobre dos monstruos" [Description of a two-headed calf followed by some reflections about two monsters], he not only recounted his findings during the dissection of the extraordinary animal but also provided an enlightened classification of "monsters," distinguishing them according to their anatomical composition and origins (Unanue 1792, 187–92).

7 This rich literary and scientific tradition reached a high point in seventeenth-century Lima with the publication of *Desvíos de la naturaleza o tratado sobre el origen de los monstruos* (1695), a book written by the surgeon Rivilla Bonet y Pueyo, in which he attempted to explain the natural and supernatural causes of phenomena such as conjoined twins and other extraordinary births and pregnancies. Larrinaga also supported his observations with quotes from Abad La Roque's *Journal de médecine* (1683), Francisco Suárez de Ribera's *Manifestación de cien secretos* (1736), and Joseph Aignan Sigaud de la Fond's *Diccionario de las maravillas de la naturaleza* (1781). Far from being a completely discredited line of inquiry, the subject of "monstrosity" had merited the philosophical and scientific attention of Enlightenment writers such as Voltaire, who devoted an article to the subject in his *Dictionnaire philosophique* (Voltaire 1829 [1764], 256–9), and the Spanish philosopher Benito Jerónimo Feijoo, who referred to it in various parts of his magnum opus *Teatro crítico universal* (Feijoo

1778, 4: 246–61, and 8: 225–56; see also Park and Daston 1981, 20–54; and Hanafi 2000).

8 He had already defended this idea in his article for the *Mercurio peruano*, "Sobre un fetus de nueve meses que sacó a una mujer por el conducto de la orina," on 3 June 1797. There he had quoted Aristotle's aphorism, "Natura doemonia est, non divina," a quotation that had also been used by Feijoo in his *Teatro crítico universal* in his discourse on the "Marvels of Nature" (Feijoo 1778, 6: 225).

9 According to Larrinaga, the monster was finally placed inside an urn and exhibited in the Hospital of Bartolomé next to the dried skeleton of a slave girl, which he used to teach students about the anatomical composition of the human body (Larrinaga 1804; Warren 2010, 69–70; Rabí Chara 2006b, 232–41). The specimen was accompanied by "an engraving of two live lizards that a woman gave birth to in Spain, one with eight feet and two tails and the other with four" (Larrinaga 1804; Rabí Chara 2006b, 239).

10 Peninsular representatives in Cádiz sought to exclude indigenous populations from the benefits of full citizenship, based in their presumed intellectual and political "minority of age." Despite this, the Cortes not only granted citizenship to American Indians but also abolished the *mita* (forced labour) and Indian tribute on 5 January 1811 and 9 November 1812, respectively (O'Phelan Godoy 2002, 178). With the indigenous population out of the equation, those most likely to be stripped of the benefit of Spanish citizenship were blacks and mulattoes, owing to their supposed inferiority. During the preliminary discussions, Agustin Arguelles, a deputy from Asturias, argued that although all social classes should be considered equal, it was not possible to grant full citizenship to those who were or had been subjected to the institution of slavery (*Diario de las discusiones y actas de las Cortes* III, 23 January 1811, 66; O'Phelan Godoy 2002, 169). Additionally, some American delegates, fearful of empowering blacks and mulattos in their home regions, supported these racially motivated arguments. Such was the case for the Peruvian delegate Morales Duárez, who represented Lima and did not hesitate to add that "the blacks are not natives, they are Africans, and as such they are excluded from the proposal, just as the mulattoes are excluded" (ibid., 61; ibid., 169).

11 It is unclear whether the author of this letter was in fact an Afro-descendant or was someone writing for *El Peruano* who pretended to pass

for one in order to support full citizenship for the *castas*. *El Peruano* was the most liberal newspaper in Lima and, as such, was frequently at odds with the administration of Viceroy Abascal. Its editors were clearly in favour of citizenship for the *castas*. On 13 March 1812 – three days after the publication of the aforementioned letter – they published a piece by Francisco Salazar, who defended granting citizenship to the *castas* as an acknowledgment of their importance in the war effort and in the general prosperity of Peru (*El Peruano*, 13 March 1812, cited in Morán Ramos 2008, 175).

12 Freedom of the press – one of the most liberal provisions of the Cortes de Cádiz – was officially announced in Lima on 18 April 1811 in the *Gaceta del gobierno* (McEvoy Carreras 2002, 836). Abascal recognized the validity of the Cortes's decree, though he immediately announced its suspension until the establishment of the Junta de censura – a committee charged with preventing revolutionary and subversive ideas from reaching the public – which finally happened in June 1811. Even so, Abascal did not hide his dissatisfaction with the newly granted freedoms, and in September of that year he informed the peninsular authorities that they "must be careful when interpreting the reach of the Law in Peru, because liberty without restrictions will increase antagonism between *peninsulares* and *criollos* and, additionally, will facilitate the infiltration of Napoleonic propaganda" (Martínez Riaza 1982, 111–12). In Peru, the decree eventually resulted in the publication of about fifteen newspapers. Morán Ramos divided the development of the Peruvian press into three stages: from 1808 to 1810, the royalist cause was supported by *Minerva peruana* (1805–10); from 1810 to 1812, the radical and critical press, which did not yet promote independence, was represented by *El Diario secreto de Lima* (1811), *El Peruano* (1811–12) and *El Satélite del peruano* (1812); and, finally, the moderate press that appeared after the promulgation of the Liberal constitution in 1812 and lasted until the return of absolutism in 1814, including *La Gaceta de Lima* (1810–12), *El Verdadero peruano* (1812–13), *El Investigador* (1813–14), *El Argos constitucional* (1813), *El Peruano liberal* (1813), and *El Clamor de la verdad* (1814) (Morán Ramos 2010, 110).

13 Bernardino Ruiz was the publisher who was in charge of printing the *Mercurio peruano* in the 1790s. His commitment to the liberal ideas that emerged after the ratification of the Cádiz Constitution is illustrated by the fact that he reprinted in Lima the declaration *Derechos y deberes del*

ciudadano, which had been printed in Cádiz in 1813. He was also the publisher of many other writers and political pamphleteers with republican tendencies (McEvoy Carreras 2002, 838).

14 Distantly related to the Inca emperor Huayna Cápac, Dionisio Inca Yupanqui was born in the 1760s. He was sent to Spain when he was still a child, in order to avoid becoming a leader of those who hoped for the return of the Incas. He was educated in the Seminario de nobles in Madrid and pursued a military career. Although he was interested in Peruvian affairs and kept channels of communication open with his homeland, much of his knowledge of his country came from indirect sources (O'Phelan Godoy 2002, 180; Villegas Páucar 2012, 1–16).

15 The census was not used for the parish elections that determined the composition of the city council, but for electing Lima's representatives to the Constitutional Cortes. Even so, it provides a good picture of the kind of problem that officials encountered when deciding who could vote in the parish elections. According to Anna, " 'Citizens with exercise' (the right to vote) were white adult male heads of households who were probably literate or semiliterate, while 'citizens without exercise' were peninsular military personnel stationed in Lima, minors, and whites who clearly fell far short of citizenship (as for example by occupation, income, or illiteracy). Ciudadanas, confusingly, were the wives and daughters of both these categories. Every viceroyalty defined citizenship on its own because it was left vague in the Constitution. The greatest distortion, however, is that the category 'Spaniards' no longer meant white, as it would have previously. The Cortes had specifically decreed that Indians and mestizos were to be called 'Spaniards,' so that category included everybody else who was not a professed regular or secular religious, a slave, or a non-national – in other words, Indians, mestizos and castas" (Anna 1975, 233).

16 *El Verdadero peruano* appeared for the first time on 22 October 1812 (Rodríguez Merino 1990, 532). In addition to Valdés, other important intellectuals of Lima such as Hipólito Unanue, José Joaquín Larría, José Baquijano y Carrillo, and Félix Devoti contributed to the newspaper as opinion writers and editors. In spite of its liberal and reformist tendencies, *El Verdadero peruano* was far less radical – and better connected to the viceregal government – than its rival *El Peruano*, a newspaper that had been edited since 1811 by Jaime Bausate y Mesa, Juan Freyre, and Miguel Eyzaguire, the last of whom frequently clashed with the Abascal

administration during the newspaper's brief existence (McEvoy Carreras 2002, 837–8).

17 At the time of Asunción's delivery in 1804, news had arrived in Lima describing the case of a peasant woman from the Duchy of Estiria (Steiermark, Austria) that seemed to support Larrinaga's conclusions. Shortly after getting married, the woman had apparently delivered a big snake along with several smaller ones and a large number of eggs. The issue was used by Larrinaga's supporters as proof that what Larrinaga had described was indeed plausible (Larrinaga 1812, 91–2), but other than that, the matter does not seem to have gone any further at the time and it was quickly forgotten. Eight years later, Larrinaga claimed in his book *Cartas históricas a un amigo* that the creatures born in Lima and Estiria were nothing less than the harbingers of the Wars of Independence in America and the Napoleonic Wars in Europe. Larrinaga argued that monsters should be understood, first of all, "as beings that exist for the honour and glory of God" and, secondly, as omens that alert mankind to "the just anger of the Heavens at the moral depravity with which man has offended the supreme Being" (Larrinaga 1812, 149). Thus, while he considered that the monster born in Lima embodied Charles IV's political mistakes, Larrinaga saw the monster born in Central Europe – an enormous viper followed by smaller snakes and many eggs – as prefiguring of "that monster of Napoleon, who resembles a reptile in his origins because of his dark and contemptible background but has nevertheless become a formidable despot throughout the world" (ibid., 150–1). This political and eschatological interpretation of a natural event must have further damaged his standing vis-à-vis Unanue, Dávalos, and Valdés. In his 1792 article "Descripción de un ternero bicípite seguida de algunas reflexiones sobre dos monstruos," Unanue had already pointed out that "in the sixteenth century people still regarded monsters with sacred terror and believed they could determine what miseries they foretold judging from their appearance alone. A two-headed monster was believed to be a clear indication of the unhappy schism brought about by the elevation of two claimants to the Sovereign Pontificate ... Centuries of darkness in which man only saw spectres and shadows and in which astrology and physics attributed the creation of monsters to the influence of eclipses and comets have been supressed by the enlightened century that we live in ... Monstrosities are now understood as simple games and caprices that Nature uses to surprise those who contemplate it,

similar to a skilled painter who sometimes abandons the ordinary rules of his Art and allows his brush to run in the direction of his divinely inspired enthusiasm" (Unanue 1792, 186–7).

18 If anything, the political situation led Valdés to put aside his liberal ideas and explore his spiritual side. In 1815 Valdés received authorization from Pope Pio VII to become a priest, since he required the Pope's permission to do so on account of his racial origins. After he received news of the papal decree he went directly to the archbishop of Lima, Bartolomé María de Las Heras, asking for permission to take the sacred vows. Proof of how quickly the racial legislation codified at Cádiz had faded into oblivion was the fact that Valdés's petition was met with strong resistance from the *cabildo catedralicio* [cathedral's council], some members of which complained that "they would soon have to share their seats in the cathedral chorus with a black man" (Lavalle n.d., 11). In light of this opposition, Valdés withdrew his petition, telling his friends that it "must not be God's will that he should become a priest and that the opposition from the ecclesiastical council was a merited punishment for his pride" (ibid.). To a certain extent, the damage to his ego was reversed when it became known that the Real Academia médico matritense [Madrid's Royal Medical Academy] had accepted him as one of its members on 19 May 1816 (Mendiburu 1890, 8: 221).

19 The situation in Lima and other Peruvian provinces substantially worsened after the royalist forces lost control of Chile in late 1817. The price of bread almost doubled, and the rise in price of nearly every basic product brought several provinces to the brink of famine. Prisons were poorly guarded, which facilitated the escape of many prisoners and created an environment of disorder and violence in the city and its surrounding regions. As if this was not enough, transatlantic commerce collapsed, despite the efforts made by the Consulate of Lima to keep the port of Callao open amidst attacks from revolutionary ships (Orrego Penagos 2009, 99).

20 As Anna has pointed out, the document containing the Declaration of Independence was left in the office of the *cabildo* secretary so that more of the public could sign it. In the end, a total of 3,504 people signed, including nearly every literate male in Lima. It is difficult to determine whether the signing of the document was a completely free act representing the collective will of Lima or whether it was a sort of "rigged

referendum" in which citizens feared the consequences of not demonstrating their support (Anna 1975, 222-44).

21 The creation of the Order of the Sun cannot be separated from San Martín's project of establishing a constitutional monarchy in Peru. The order was created "to honour the year of Peruvian 'regeneration' and to pass to posterity the names of the principals in the independence movement. The highest ranking political and military advisers, including Hipólito Unanue, were knighted as 'Founders,' and they enjoyed the privilege of being treated as nobility, of being addressed as 'Honourable,' and of wearing a white sash that distinguished the members of the order. There were two additional classes, 'Beneméritos' and 'Associates,' but unlike the 'Founders,' their titles were not hereditary" (Woodham 1964, 274).

22 According to Lavalle, who cites Manuel de Odriozola's *Documentos literarios del Perú*, Valdés presented a medical essay to the members of the Sociedad patriótica on 12 July 1822 (Lavalle n.d., 16; Odriozola 1877, 450). Unfortunately, neither Lavalle nor Odriozola provide information about the topic of Valdés's presentation. The members of the organization may have been more interested in debating politics than medicine. As Woodham points out, the Sociedad patriótica "functioned as a literary and debating club and published a newspaper, *El sol del Perú*, and in these characteristics resembled the Amantes del País society of the 1790s. But the president, Monteagudo, rigged the discussions so that the proponents of monarchism could have a forum, and thereby gave the society a stronger political emphasis. Although the members considered other topics, such as the causes that had retarded independence in Lima, they spent most of their time debating the merits of monarchical and republican forms of government" (Woodham 1964, 274-5).

23 José Mariano de la Riva Agüero y Sánchez Boquete (1783-1858) was a major figure during the Wars of Independence in Peru and the first to be designated as President of the Republic. Born in Lima into a wealthy aristocratic family, Riva Agüero played a pivotal role in the groups that advocated independence from Spain in the 1810s. As war broke out, he joined those who supported the invasion led by José de San Martín, who made him prefect of Lima in 1821, a position he used to consolidate his influence. On 28 February 1823, Congress elected Riva Agüero as President of the Republic after the revolutionary army forced it to dissolve

the Suprema Junta Gubernativa created by San Martín in 1822 following a series of military setbacks. However, Riva Agüero's tenure in office was short. The occupation of Lima by the Spaniards on 19 June 1823 led to a government crisis and to the Peruvian Congress's decision to grant extraordinary powers to the Venezuelan general Antonio José de Sucre, stripping Riva Agüero of his authority. Riva Agüero reacted by decreeing the dissolution of Congress on 19 July 1823. Bolívar's support of Sucre, the constitution of a new congress, and the election of Torre Tagle as provisional president of Peru further isolated Riva Agüero, who tried to reaffirm his position by negotiating a truce with the Spanish forces. This was not to be. He was detained by his own officers on 25 November 1823 and sent into exile. He returned to Peru in 1831, and in 1836 became provisional president of the Republic of North Peru, which was part of the Peru-Bolivian Confederation created by Bolivian president Andrés de Santa Cruz. Santa Cruz's defeat at the battle of Yungay in 1839 put an end to the confederation and to the political career of Riva Agüero. He died in Lima on 25 May 1858. For more information about his life and work see Bronner (1956) and Jiménez Borja (1962).

CHAPTER FOUR

1 Born in Lima on 29 September 1766, Tafur had become chair of Método de Medicina at the University of San Marcos in 1798 and chair of Vísperas in 1814 (ix, xiii). In addition to his role as substitute protomédico, a role that he had also played from 1814 to 1817 while Unanue was in Spain, he was also made principal of the University of San Marcos and chair of Prima de Medicina in 1826 (Lastres 1943, i–xix; Mendiburu 1890, 8: 7–8; Gittinger 1945, 316).

2 They argued that not just Peru but Lima itself constituted a distinct pathological environment (Warren 2004, 31). The corollary was clear: while doctors should make every effort to keep informed of the latest developments in the field, epidemic illnesses had to be studied and treated according to the observations and methods developed *in situ* and not according to what European theorists may have found to be more appropriate for their own countries. In this regard, few things of substance changed in Peruvian medicine in the late 1820s. Unanue's highly influ-

ential *El clima de Lima*, which he wrote between 1799 and 1805, was still the reference book for most general medical issues in early republican Peru.

3 Valdés considered Blanco's case representative of patients who attributed their health to Dorotea's remedies rather than to the effects of their doctors' prescriptions. As Blanco's condition worsened – he was suffering from dysentery – the doctors who oversaw him decided that bloodletting was the best remedy, "judging by the fact that he was suffering of an inflammatory illnesss" (*Mercurio peruano*, 18 February 1831, 1). Some members of his family protested, concerned that Blanco was about to die, but the doctors replied that his situation was not so serious. After having been given this procedure twice that day and once again on the next, Blanco recovered, but he credited his recovery not to the beneficial effects of bloodletting but to the remedies clandestinely administered by Dorotea, an opinion that Valdés contemptuously dismissed (ibid.).

4 The Anti-Svadel published a second text a few days later, expanding some of the ideas that had appeared in his first letter. Among them, he emphasized the connection between the Protomedicato and Peru's colonial past: "The Spanish government, which was essentially monarchical and despotic, did the right thing in establishing the Protomedicato as a tribunal full of privileges, restrictive laws, and penalties. This fitted with its plans for absolute domination aimed at breaking up society, creating privileged institutions, and – with the cooperation of local and provincial police – monopolizing science, industry, knowledge, the arts, and everything that belonged to all men by nature without any limitation. This must not be allowed in a Republic with a representative form of government in which the principles of equality, individual security, freedom, and property are deified and occupy a prominent place in the altar of its Constitution" (*Mercurio peruano*, 9 March 1831, 3). This text is reproduced *verbatim* on page 19 of the *Defensa hecha a favor de doña Dorotea Salguero* (1831), which is signed by Manuel Cayetano Loyo, himself a doctor and a legislative representative (*diputado*) from Arequipa, who participated in the founding of the Colegio de la Independencia of that city and in the writing of the Constitution of 1826 (See *Constitución para la República peruana* (1826, 54). Paradoxically, Cayetano Loyo did not extend the defence of his radical liberalism concerning medicine to other issues. In the controversial issue of tobacco, he

argued in favour of restricting its trade because of his conviction that "free commerce allows for the limitations that best suit the Republic" (Cayetano de Loyo n.d., 8).

5 Valdés considered Dorotea the latest example of a long succession of folk healers, such as Villafani – who claimed to be able to predict future illnesses by taking the pulse of his patients – and Father Matraya – who caused a great deal of harm in Lima with Leroy's Panquimagogo (*Mercurio peruano*, 3 March 1831, 3). Valdés argued that even if Dorotea was as good a herbalist as her supporters contended, she was still not qualified as a physician. Physicians were supposed to know the properties of the remedies they used and the illnesses for which they could be prescribed. They should also be informed about other physical and moral variables that frequently explained why a certain medicine did not work for all patients suffering from the same illness. For Valdés, medicine's arcane secrets were revealed only after careful study and observation of the language through which the body expressed itself, and this could not be understood by a simple folk healer.

6 Some of them even included *ad hominem* attacks on Valdés and the protomédico Miguel Tafur. A reader who identified himself simply as "El sacerdote agradecido" (the grateful priest) denounced Valdés as "sacrilegious, envious, and greedy" for attending daily mass while bearing false testimony against a humble woman who, "in her treatments, performs nothing less than works of charity" (*Mercurio peruano*, 14 April 1831, 2). Valdés's answer was to forgive the insults directed at him while reminding "the grateful priest" of a passage from the Bible (Luke 6:13): "Judge not and you will not be judged. Condemn not and you will not be condemned. Forgive and you will be forgiven. By the grace of God, I pardon you one thousand and one times everything you have said, published, and thought of me, so that my sins can also be pardoned; and I will pray that He does not punish you as He threatens to do with those who judge their peers" (*Mercurio peruano*, No. 1078, 15 April 1831, 2).

7 At the beginning of her case, Dorotea submitted an appeal to the Peruvian Congress denouncing what she considered a biased trial. She asked the political representatives to let her continue practising medicine and to allow citizens to be healed by whomever they chose, without the intervention of the Protomedicato general de la República, but it is not clear what happened with the documentation. A letter submitted to the *Mercurio peruano* complained that "the briefs presented by Dorotea

Salguero were mislaid with the greatest ease" and wondered how many people – including "some subordinate employees of the secretary of the Congress" – might have taken part in the destruction of her documents (*Mercurio peruano*, 15 March 1831, 4). To counter such insinuations, several congressional employees published a long letter detailing the petitions submitted by Dorotea, all of which were filed in 1827 and 1828. Moreover, they stated that the petitions had been rejected and that the resolutions concerning her case had always been at her disposal in the congressional archives (ibid.). Apparently, Dorotea submitted her petition once again in a letter signed on 16 June 1831, which included a copy of her *Defensa* (*Defensa* 1831, 50–61). It is not known, however, whether the issue ended up being debated by Congress or, as in the previous cases, the dossier was lost or once again rejected.

8 Apart from the Protomedicato, the two most important institutions charged with overseeing the practice of medicine in republican Peru were the Dirección general de beneficencia and the Junta de sanidad. Created in October 1825, the Dirección general de beneficencia was charged with the supervision of Peruvian hospitals, which had been in decline on account of the economic problems suffered by the religious brotherhoods that had traditionally been in charge of them. The office lasted only until 1834, when it was supplanted by more regionally oriented Sociedades de beneficencia (Bustios Romani 2004, 308–10). As for the Juntas de sanidad, they were created by a supreme decree on 1 September 1826, under the government of Andrés de Santa Cruz. They were charged with overseeing all matters of public health in the republic, along with establishing other Juntas de sanidad at the regional and municipal levels (*Colección de leyes 1862*, 8:, 323–7). The composition of the *junta*, however, still allowed the Protomédico general de la República to have a defining role. It consisted of six members: the prefect of the Department of Lima, the Protomédico general, another doctor, a chemist, and two city neighbours who were to be married landowners but not businessmen. The Protomédico general was supposed to preside over the *junta* whenever the prefect could not attend (*Colección de leyes 1862*, 8: 324). While extraordinary powers were given to the Junta de sanidad, the institution was largely ineffectual because of lack of funding and the frequency of political changes in Peru. Therefore, the office of the Protomedicato exercised *de facto* control over matters that should have been discussed at the *juntas* or even at the Dirección general de beneficencia

(Bustios Romani 2004, 254–9). This situation persisted until the creation of the Junta directiva de medicina on 30 December 1848, which marked the end of the protomedicato (Bustios Romani 2004, 302).

9 In Valdés's opinion, the disease had found fertile ground in a population already weakened by "successive revolutions, which have caused the population a great deal of bitterness and sorrow" (Valdés 1835a, 7). The unusual fluctuations in temperature and humidity experienced in Lima during the previous years had also contributed to the increased number of outbreaks. The effects of these fluctuations may have been made considerably worse by other natural phenomena, such as the earthquake that shook Lima on 30 March 1828, which Valdés suspected of having "altered and noticeably spoiled our atmosphere" (ibid.). To make things worse, the poor quality of the food consumed in the capital, especially the flour used to bake bread, had increased the frequency of gastro-intestinal problems and contributed to the spread of the disease.

10 Apparently, it was not the first time that Valdés had saved this patient's life. The first occasion was during the Dorotea Salguero affair. As he put it, he was forced to seek the help of Dorotea "on account of the few relations I had in this country and her fame as folk healer, and I am sure I would have died as a result of her prescribed diet for dysentery – broths, pig's meat, milk, and chocolate – if you [Dr Valdés] had not saved me" (*El Rejenerador*, 16 June 1835, 1–2).

11 Archibald Smith had arrived in Peru in 1826 to work as a doctor for the Anglo-Pasco Peruvian Mining Company, a British firm dedicated to the extraction of silver in Cerro de Pasco, an important mine in central Peru. The company went bankrupt just a year after Smith's arrival. After a failed attempt to settle in the valley of Huanuco, Smith moved to Lima in 1830. Once there, he obtained the backing of influential figures from the British community, soon becoming ward physician at the Hospital de Santa Ana and medical adviser at the Hospital de San Andrés, where he cared for British and American citizens and sailors arriving in Peru (Lossio 2006, 834–5).

12 Joaquín Jiménez, the controller at the Hospital de Santa Ana, confirmed Smith's accusations in a letter published in *El Rejenerador* two days later. According to Jiménez, there had been a noticeable decrease in the number of deaths since the British doctor took over the department in charge of dysenteric patients compared with the hundreds who had died when

it was under the charge of Valdés. He attributed this difference to the protomédico's proclivity to prescribe bloodletting and never-ending diets to treat the illness (*El Rejenerador*, supplt., 21 July 1835, 2). Valdés later refuted the hospital controller's account and Smith's allegations as slanderous. He also pointed out that he was at the helm of that medical department for only four months, during which only two patients died of dysentery (Valdés 1835b, 5–6).

13 According to Johnson, the best remedy for curing dysentery was to to give mercury "in comparatively small doses, either alone, or combined with an anodyne, or with an anodyne and diaphoretic [which is preferable], in such a manner, that, from 24 to 36 or 48 grains of calomel, according to the urgency of the symptoms, may be exhibited, in divided portions, at three, four, or six-hour intervals, during the course of the day and night. In the same space of time, from two to four grains of opium, and from ten to fifteen grains of antimonial powder, may with advantage be administered, in combination with the calomel. One or two doses, at least, should be given, before a laxative is prescribed; and an ounce of castor oil is the best medicine I can recommend for the latter purpose. It will often bring away hardened fecal, or vitiated bilious accumulations, when the irritability of the intestines is previously allayed by the calomel and opium; and it will, in that manner, soothe the tormina and tenesmus. But although it may be repeated every day, it is never to interrupt the progress of the main remedy" (Johnson 1815 [1813], 271).

14 The first case in which Valdés and Smith worked together concerned a rich patient from Ica who suspected he had an aneurism. He therefore travelled to Lima and met with the most distinguished doctors of the city to discuss the appropriate treatment. Smith and another English doctor named Kinston supported the patient's self-diagnosis of an aneurism, which Valdés adamantly opposed. The majority of the *junta* supported Valdés's conclusion, which the English doctors found exceedingly annoying. According to Valdés, the patient later thanked him for saving his life. Valdés and Smith met again soon afterwards to deal with the case of the Mexican ambassador, José Joaquín Mora, who had developed a grave case of dysentery. Again Valdés and Smith proposed different treatments, but it was Valdés who convinced his colleagues to follow his prescription of bloodletting, after which the patient recovered (Valdés 1835b, 1–2). The final encounter between the two men took place two

months later. It involved the head of the Nazarene Order in Peru, Manuel Soriano, who had fallen ill with an acute fever. Smith and another doctor were in charge of his treatment. According to Valdés, after the patient had already lost all feeling in his body due to the fever, Smith and his colleague put blistering plaster on his legs and head and bottles of warm water on the soles of his feet that were so hot that they burnt his skin. Since the patient gave no sign of recovery, Smith left him for dead after three days. His family then called Valdés, even though they expected the patient to die at any moment. Valdés suggested to start bleeding him from the foot that very night. Four days later the supposedly hopeless patient had fully recovered (ibid.).

15 As mentioned in the preface of this book, Smith concluded his overview of Peruvian medicine with a racial generalization that he did not articulate during his controversy with Valdés but that had "consequences of vital interest to society" and may have influenced his perception of his adversary. According to Smith, the degeneration of medicine in Lima could largely be attributed to the fact that most physicians "were raised from among the genuine black, or other more or less crossed Ethiopian castes, to whom, as is affirmed by Ayanque at page 43 of his celebrated satire, titled *Lima por dentro y fuera*, the healing art in all its branches, and especially surgery, was almost entirely intrusted" (Smith 1839, 179). As doctors and viceroys had done in the mid-eighteenth century, Smith introduced the racial argument as an explanation for the underdeveloped state of Peruvian medicine in the decades following independence. Archibald Smith was not the only foreigner to lament the state of Peruvian medicine and to blame it on the racial origins of Peruvian doctors. Johan Jakob von Tschudi, a Swiss naturalist who spent four years in Peru in the late 1830s, observed with disdain, that "Most of the physicians in Lima are mulattoes; but they are remarkable only for their ignorance, as they receive neither theoretical nor clinical instruction. Nevertheless, they enjoy the full confidence of the public, who rank the ignorant native far above the educated foreigner" (Von Tschudi 1854, 83).

16 Valdés's difficult relationship with foreign doctors did not begin in the 1830s. As early as 1818, he was involved in a controversy with Joaquín Solano, a Spanish physician in the Royal Navy, over the use of emetic tartar and an antimonial mixture in the treatment of bilious fever and diarrhea. Valdés criticized those physicians in Lima who, "fascinated by a few modern authors," recommended such remedies. He advocated lim-

iting their use only to "doctors who have been proved capable of discerning the circumstances that require their application in the few occasions that required it" (Valdés 1818, 139; see also Solano 1818, 184–9). Even if remedies such as emetic tartar had proved useful in Europe, Valdés argued that they might not be so effective in Lima since, in his opinion, medicines must be tailored to the needs of specific countries. Valdés strongly recommended using local remedies instead: "lemonades, cream, or tamarinds in natural water or a broth, and, for nourishment, a porridge made of flour, corn, or rice with some acidic juice" (Valdés 1818, 139).

17 The regulations also established guidelines to teach students how to write a patient's clinical history (*Reglamento* 1862 [1840], título 7, art. 32 and Art. 33). Valdés proposed that the best of these clinical histories should be printed and archived as "the most useful treasure for the practice of medicine and the surest way to discover those who will become the best doctors" (ibid., título 7, art. 38).

18 Peruvian historians have dismissed Valdés's regulations as the work of an old man who was "stubbornly opposed to abandoning scholastic medicine" and have praised the reforms undertaken by Heredia (Bustios Romani 2004, 295). While there were not significant changes in the administrative direction of the school, Heredia's regulations did help to modernize the curriculum more than those proposed by Valdés. The school incorporated the study of chemistry, natural history, and legal medicine. In their first year, students would study anatomy, skeletology, epidemiology, splanchnology, chemistry, and mineralogy; in their second year, arterial angiology, veins and lymphs, neurology, pathological anatomy, physiology and hygiene, botany, and again chemistry; in their third year, pathology and general therapeutics, medical material, and zoology; in their fourth year, medical nosography, internal and clinical medicine, medical material, and the art of prescribing; in the fifth year, medical nosography, legal medicine, surgical institutions, topographical anatomy, and again internal medicine; and, during their final year, surgical institutions, external and clinical medicine, legal medicine, and obstetrics. The curriculum also included the study of philosophy and mathematics as complementary courses for the students. Heredia also established recommendations concerning the way in which each discipline should be taught. For chemistry, students had to learn organic and inorganic chemistry without losing sight of its applications to pharma-

cology. For medical material, he stressed the utility of knowing and studying indigenous remedies. Heredia mantained that legal medicine should not be limited to forensics but should also deal with the study of the role of medicine in politics and legislation. Even though his proposal departed significantly from that articulated by Valdés, Heredia valued Valdés's suggestion of preserving the best clinical histories to serve as an example for future doctors and as a means of researching the illnesses most commonly experienced in Peru (*Colección de leyes* 1862 [1843], 9: 199–209).

CONCLUSION

1 Tomás Jacinto Cipolleti, Master of the Dominican Order, was the main figure at the Vatican who advocated the beatificacion of Martín de Porres and Juan Macías. For his part, Lázaro Balaguer y Cubillas lobbied from Lima and sent Porres's and Macías's relics to Rome, along with a letter to the Pope in which he expressed his wish that "the Holy Father declare those two venerable servants of God, Friar Juan Macías and Friar Martín de Porres, not only as Blessed but also as Saints, since this will comfort both our Order and the whole of the Peruvian Republic" (Valdés 1863 [1840], 187). Balaguer y Cubilla's interest in the beatification of Martín de Porres – and in that of Juan Macías, who was beatified on the same occasion – went beyond the simple desire to see two fellow Dominicans elevated to the altars. For him, as for the Order of Preachers in general, it was a way to recover from the trauma suffered during independence, when the Dominican Province of San Juan Bautista del Perú "was immersed in the most intense crisis in its history, being reduced to only three monasteries as result of a decree issued by the republican government on 23 March 1822" ("Reseña" 2012).

2 Lavalle attributes this ode to José Manuel Valdés, although he dates its composition to 1828 instead of 1822 (Lavalle 1863, 463). There is no doubt that this is a mistake, given that the document clearly states 1822 as its date of publication (Valdés 1822, 14). The issue of freedom of religion was discussed by Peru's Constituent Congress in 1822, and it was roundly rejected in the Constitution of 1823. *Appletons' Cyclopeida of American Biography* (1889, 223) also attributes this work to Valdés.

3 The description of Martín de Porres's passing, which took place on the night of 3 November 1639, followed the archetypical narrative expected

of a future saint. After succumbing to a long agony, during which he was able to resist the temptations of the Devil, one of the friars who had been present all along questioned the body of Porres: "How, my brother Fray Martín, do you appear so stiff when the dawn is approaching and the whole city is waiting to see you and praise God and his wonders? Ask Him that, using His power, He makes your body docile and supple once again"; then, suddenly, the body became "softer and more docile and agreeable than when the Servant of God was alive" (Medina 1673, 217). Those who attended his burial testified that the body "gave off a heavenly odour that captivated those present to the point that they were unable to compare it with any earthly aroma" (ibid., 218). When years later the decision to remove the corpse from the crypt was made, the friars in charge of the excavation testified that they found the bones "covered with living flesh and blood, as if they had just been buried," and giving off "such a fragrant odour of roses that suspended and pleased the sense of smell of those who were there" (ibid., 232).

4 Valdés readily conceded that there were events, for which science could not produce a viable explanation, but they were a clear minority and not always connected to medicine. Among them, Valdés cited Martín de Porres's ability to plant hundreds of olive trees in just one day – which germinated immediately thereafter – as well as his power to divert the flooded Rimac River, which threatened to engulf Lima, using only three stones and the invocation of the Holy Trinity (Valdés 1863 [1840], 125–6). He also gave credence to some of the saint's miraculous cures, such as when Martín de Porres instantly healed a fellow friar's gangrenous leg with just a prayer and by laying his hands upon him or when he was able to resurrect a man that doctors had already declared dead (ibid., 127). Valdés even accepted some of the reports that claimed that Martín de Porres continued performing cures after his death, including the case of a woman who was cured of a painful abscess by just spreading soil taken from the saint's grave over it (ibid., 182).

5 No less than five constitutions were drafted between 1821 and 1844, a period when the country had over fifteen different heads of state (Bustio Romani 2004, 210). One of the latest episodes in the Peruvian political drama was the defeat of Andrés de Santa Cruz, President of Bolivia and Supreme Protector of Perú, in the battle of Yungay in January 1839, which put an end to the confederation between the two countries.

~

Bibliography

ARCHIVES

AAL   Archivo arzobispal de Lima (Lima, Peru)
AGI   Archivo general de Indias (Seville, Spain)
AGN   Archivo general de la Nación (Lima, Peru)
AHN   Archivo histórico nacional (Madrid, Spain)
AML   Archivo municipal de Lima (Lima, Peru)
BNP   Biblioteca nacional de Perú (Lima, Peru)

HISTORICAL SOURCES

Almeida, Teodoro de. 1792. *Recreaciones filosóficas, o Diálogo sobre la filosofía natural para instrucción de personas curiosas que no han frecuentado las aulas.* Vol. 4. Madrid: Imprenta Real

"Apéndice de la sociedad." 1791. *Mercurio peruano* 47 (12 June): 108–11

Appletons' Cyclopedia of American Biography. 1889. Vol. 6, ed. Grant Wilson, James Fiske and John Fiske. New York: D. Appleton and Company

Aristotle. 1831. *De divinatione per somnum.* In *Aristotelis Opera.* Vol. 3, ed. Academia Regia Borusica. Berolini: Georgium Reimerum.

Astruc, Jean. 1763. *Tractatus de morbis mulierum.* Venice: Niccolo Pezzana

Ayanque, Simón (pseudonym of Esteban Terralla y Landa). 1798. *Lima por dentro y fuera en consejos económicos, saludables, políticos y morales que da un amigo a otro con motivo de querer dejar la ciudad de México por pasar a la de Lima*. Madrid: Imprenta de Villalpando

Bottoni, Federico. 1723. *Evidencia de la circulación de la sangre*. Lima: Imprenta de la Calle de Palacio

Bravo de Lagunas y Castilla, Pedro Joseph. 1761. *Discurso histórico-jurídico del origen, fundación, reedificación, derechos y exenciones del hospital de San Lázaro de Lima*. Lima: Oficina de los Huérfanos

Bueno de la Rosa, Hipólito. 1764. *Causa médico criminal que en este real protomedicato del Perú han seguido los profesores de la facultad de medicina contral los cirujanos, farmacéuticos, phlebotómicos, etc. sobre contenerlos en los términos de sus respectivas profesiones*. Lima: En la Oficina de la Calle de la Encarnación

Buffon, Georges Louis Leclerc, Comte de. 1791. *Natural History, General and Particular*. Trans. William Smellie. 9 vols. London: A. Strahan and T. Cadell. [Translation of *Histoire naturelle générale et particulière*. Paris: Imprimerie Royale, 1749–67]

Calancha, Antonio de la. 1639. *Coronica moralizada de la Orden de San Agustín en el Perú*. Barcelona: Por Pedro Lacavallería en la Librería

Calero y Moreira, Jacinto. 1790. "Prospecto del papel intitulado *Mercurio peruano de historia, literatura y noticias públicas*." Lima: En la Imprenta Real de los Niños Expósitos

Cangiamila, Francesco Emanuello. 1745. *Embriologia sacra, ovvero dell'uffizio de'sacerdoti, medici, e superiori, circa l'etherna salute de' bambini racchiusi nell'utero*. Palermo: Francesco Valenza

Causa médico criminal que en este Real Protomedicato del Perú han seguido los profesores de la facultad médica contra los cirujanos, farma-céuticos, flebotómicos, etc. 1764. Lima: En la oficina de la Calle de la Encarnación

Cayetano de Loyo, Manuel. 1827. *Voto particular del diputado que suscribe sobre el restablecimiento de la renta de tabacos en el Perú*. Lima: n.p.

Cerdán y Pontero, Ambrosio. 1794. "Progresos y estado actual de la *Sociedad de Amantes del País*." *Mercurio peruano* 329–332 (27 February–9 March): 135–65

Cobo, Bernabé. 1882 [1639]. *Historia de la fundación de Lima*. Lima: Imprenta Liberal.

Colección de leyes, decretos y ordenes publicadas en el Peru desde su independencia en el año de 1821 hasta 31 de diciembre de 1830. 1832. Vol. 3. Lima: J. Masías

Colección de leyes, decretos y ordenes publicadas en el Peru desde el año de 1821 hasta 31 de diciembre de 1859. 1861–1872. 16 vols. Lima: F. Bailly

Colección de los discursos que pronunciaron los señores diputados de América contra el artículo 22 del proyecto de constitución. Ilustrado con algunas notas interesantes por los españoles pardos de esta capital. 1812. Lima: Bernardino Ruiz en la Imprenta de los Huérfanos

Constituciones y ordenanzas antiguas, añadidas y modernas de la Real universidad y estudio general de San Marcos de la ciudad de los Reyes del Perú. 1735. Lima: Felix de Saldaña y Flores

Constituciones y ordenanzas del Hospital Real de Santa Ana de Lima. 1778. Lima: En la Imprenta de los Huérfanos

Constitución para la república peruana. 1826. Lima: J. Masías

Constitución política de la monarquía española: Promulgada en Cádiz a 19 de marzo de 1812. 1820. Madrid: Imprenta que fue de García; Imprenta nacional

Covarrubias, Sebastián de. 1610. *Emblemas morales.* Madrid: Luis Sánchez

Dávalos, José Manuel. 1787. *Specimen academicum de morbis nonnullis Limae grassantibus ipsorumque therapeia* [*On some common illnesses in Lima and their therapy*]. Montpellier: Apud Joannem-Franciscum Picot

– 1810. *Alegato que en la oposición a la cátedra de método de medicina de la Real universidad de san marcos dijo el D.D. José Manuel Dávalos, graduado en las universidades de Montpeller y en la de S. Marcos de Lima y Socio de la Académica Médica de París, el día cinco de Junio de mil setecientos noventa y ocho.* Cádiz: Por D. Nicolás Gómez de Requena, 1810

– 1815. *Arenga que en el besamanos del 30 de mayo de 1815 tenido en celebridad de los felices años de S.M. pronunció en nombre del colegio de San Fernando el Dr. D. José Manuel Dávalos.* Lima: n.p.

– 1818. "Informe que dio el doctor Dávalos a la Junta Central sobre el estado actual de la vacuna." *Gaceta del gobierno de Lima* 59 (26 September): 494–7

– 1821. "Testamento de José Manuel Dávalos." AGN, Protocolos notariales (siglo XIX), Escribano Juan Pio de Espinosa. 22 October. 354r–357v

Dávila Condemarín, José. 1854. *Bosquejo histórico de la fundación de la insigne universidad mayor de San Marcos de Lima.* Lima: Imprenta de Eusebio Aranda

Defensa hecha a favor de Da. Dorotea Salguero en la causa criminal que se la ha formado a moción del protomedicato por haber curado contra sus prohibiciones y las del juez de primera instancia, en recurso a la representación nacional. 1831. Lima: Imprenta de José María Masías

Diario de las discusiones y actas de las Cortes. 1811–1813. 18 vols. Cádiz: En la Imprenta Real

Dios López, Juan de. 1785. *Compendio anatómico. Part 3: Esplanchnología. De la naturaleza y circunstancias de todas las vísceras o entrañas contenidas en las tres cavidades.* Vol. 2. Madrid: Imprenta del Consejo de Indias

Espíritu de los mejores diarios literarios que se publican en Europa. 1787 (July). Madrid: n.p.

Eyzaguirre, Eugenio. 1834. *Concertatio medica de dysenteria quam pro gradu licentiatus obtinendo auspice Deo, et Praeside D. D. Emmanuele Valdes, primae madicinae exedrae moderatore, et Reipublicae peruanae Archiatro.* Lima: Imprenta de J. Masías.

Feijoo, *Teatro crítico universal.* 1778–79. 8 vols. Madrid: Por don Joaquín Ibarra

Fernández Morejón, Antonio. 1842–47. *Historia bibliográfica de la medicina española.* 5 vols. Madrid: Viuda de Jordán e hijos

Figueroa, Juan de. 1660. *Opúsculo de astrología en medicina, y de los términos, y partes de la Astronomía necesarias para el uso de ella.* Lima: n.p.

Foderé, Françoise-Emmanuel. 1813. *Traité de médicine-légale et d'hygiène publique ou de police de santé.* 6 vols. Paris: De l'impremerie de Mame

Fox, Richard Hingston. 1901. *William Hunter, Anatomist, Physician, Obstetrician (1718–1783), with Notices of His Friends Cullen, Smellie, Fothergill, and Baillie.* London: H.K. Lewis

Fragoso, Juan. 1627 [1586]. *Cirugía universal, ahora nuevamente añadida con todas las dificultades y cuestiones pertenecientes a las materias que se trata.* Madrid: Por la Viuda de Alcaso Martia

Fuentes, Manuel Atanasio. 1985 [1867]. *Lima: Apuntes históricos, descriptivos, estadísticos y de costumbres.* Facsimile. Lima: Fondo del libro, Banco Industrial del Perú

– 1866a. *Lima, or Sketches of the Capital of Peru, Historical, Statistical, Administrative, Commercial, and Moral.* London: Trübner & Co.

– 1866b. *Aletazos del murciélago.* Paris: Ad Lainé and J. Harvard

– 1875. *Lecciones de jurisprudencia médica.* Lima: Imprenta del Estado

– 1877. *Catecismo de economía política.* Lima: Imprenta del Estado

Gago de Vadillo, Pedro. 1692 [1630] *Luz de la verdadera cirujía.*
Pamplona: Juan Micol

González Laguna, Francisco. 1781. *El zelo sacerdotal para con los niños no-nacidos.* Lima: Imprenta de los niños expósitos

Gregory XVI, Pope. 1839. *In supremo apostolatus.* Papal Encyclicals Online (accessed 5 April 2012). http://www.papalencyclicals.net/Greg16/g16sup.htm

Gumilla, Joseph. 1791. *Historia natural, civil y geográfica de las naciones situadas en las riveras del río Orinoco.* Vol. 2. Barcelona: Carlos Gibert y Tutó

Haënke, Tadeo [Thaddäus]. 1901. *Descripción del Perú.* Lima: Imprenta de "El Lucero"

Herrera, J.D. 1843. "Servicios hechos a la medicina peruana por el doctor Valdés." *El Comercio* (Lima) 1225 (13 July): 3

Hidalgo de Agüero, Bartolomé. 1604. *Thesoro de la verdadera cirugía y vía particular contra la común opinión.* Seville: Francisco Pérez

"Historia de la sociedad académica de amantes del País y principios del Mercurio peruano." 1791. *Mercurio peruano* 7 (23 January): 49–56

Indice general, alfabético y por fechas de los 6 tomos de la colección de leyes, decretos y órdenes publicadas en el Perú desde su independencia. 1845. Lima: J. Masías

Johnson, James. 1815 [1813]. *The Influence of Tropical Climates on European Constitutions.* London: J. Callow

Konetzke, Richard, ed. 1958. *Colección de documentos para la historia social de Hispanoamérica.* 5 vols. Madrid: CSIC

Laborde, Alexandre de. *Itinéraire descriptif de l'Espagne.* 1809. 5 vols. Paris: Nicolle & Lenormant

Larrinaga, José Pastor de. 1791. *Apología de los cirujanos del Perú.* Granada: Imprenta de D. Antonio Zea

– 1792a. "Sobre un fetus de nueve meses que sacó a una mujer por el conducto de la orina el año de 1779." *Mercurio peruano* 147–9 (31 May & 3–7 June): 65–84

– 1792b. "En que se trata si una mujer se puede convertir en hombre." *Mercurio peruano* 167–8 (9–12 August): 230–43

– 1792c. "Introducción a la historia de los Incas del Perú." *Mercurio peruano* 176 (9 September): 17–25

– 1792d. "Disertación de cirugía sobre un aneurisma del labio inferior." *Mercurio peruano* 197–8 (22–25 November): 189–212

– 1793a. "Sucesión cronológica de los señores gobernadores, presidentes, virreyes y capitanes generales después de los Incas del Perú." *Mercurio peruano* 227 (7 March): 159–66

– 1793b. "Carta remitida a la sociedad en contestación de la crítica que se imprimió en el *Mercurio peruano* del día 24 de febrero, número 224." *Mercurio peruano* 246 (12 May): 26–35

– 1802. *Ordenanzas de la sociedad patriótica del Monte Pío de los cirujanos del Perú, aprobada por este Superior Gobierno y Real acuerdo de justicia en 12 de marzo de 1800 y Discurso con que se hizo la apertura de esta sociedad a todos los cirujanos, la tarde del día 22 de abril siendo presidente y juez conservador de turno, el señor Márquez de Santa María, alcalde de primer voto del M.L. c. y R. de esta muy noble y muy leal ciudad de Lima.* Lima: Imprenta de la Casa Real de niños expósitos

– 1804. *Descripción de un esqueleto que se ha de colocar el día 24 de agosto de este año de 1804, en el Real Hospital de San Bartolomé, por los practicantes de cirugía baxo la dirección del protocirujano José Pastor Larrinaga.* Lima: n.p.

– 1812. *Cartas históricas a un amigo o Apología del pichón palomino.* Lima: Imprenta de los Huérfanos

– 1814. "Nota de José Pastor Pastor Larrinaga al Cabildo: Octavas dedicas a Fernando VII 'El grande.'" AML, Sección Expedientes y particulares 1796–1839, doc. 20. 6 September

Lavalle, José Antonio de. 1863. *El doctor don José Manuel Valdés: Apuntes sobre su vida y sus obras.* Lima: Tipografía nacional

– n.d. *El doctor don José Manuel Valdés: Apuntes sobre su vida y sus obras.* BNP, Colección Zegarra, XZ-v.21-f.2 9 (handwritten)

Lequanda, Joseph Ignacio. 1793. "Descripción geográfica de la ciudad y partido de Trujillo." *Mercurio peruano* 247–54 (16 May–9 June): 44–97

– 1794. "Discurso sobre el destino que debe darse a la gente vaga que tiene Lima." *Mercurio peruano* 325–8 (13–23 February): 103–32

Leroy, Louis. 1817. *La médecine naturelle et curative, ou La purgation dirigée contre la cause des maladies.* Paris: Nicolas-Vaucluse

Libro primero de Cabildos de Lima. 1888. 3 vols, ed. Enrique Torres Saldamando, Pablo Patrón, and Nicalor Boloña. Paris: Imprimerie P. Dupont

Luna Pizarro, Francisco Javier. 1858. "Arenga pronunciada en el besamanos del 30 de mayo de 1820, día del Rey nuestro Señor, por el rector del Real Colegio de San Fernando, Dr. D. Francisco Javier de Luna Pizarro." In *Memorias y documentos para la historia de la independencia del Perú y causas del mal éxito que ha tenido ésta.* Vol. 2, 124–6 Paris: Librería de Garnier

Martínez, Martín. 1752. *Anatomía completa del hombre con todos los hallazgos, nuevas doctrinas y observaciones raras hasta el tiempo presente, y muchas advertencias necesarias para la cirugía.* Madrid: Por los herederos de don Miguel Francisco Rodríguez

Matraya, Juan. 1825a. *Defensa de la medicina curativa y lícita administración de su único remedio nombrado panquimagogo por cualquiera instruido en su dirección práctica aunque sea clérigo o religioso.* Lima: Imprenta administrada por Julian González

– 1825b. *Triunfo de la medicina curativa de Mr. Leroy, sobre la paliativa, dirigido al Sr. Dr. D. Miguel Tafur, protomédico de Lima.* Lima: Imprenta de La Libertad

– 1826. *El Anti-Philathros, a los SS. promédico de Lima, Dr. D. Miguel Tafur y compañeros.* Lima: Imprenta de la Libertad

Medina, Bernardo de. 1673. *Vida prodigiosa del venerable siervo de Dios fr. Martín de Porras.* Lima: En la imprenta de Juan de Quevedo y Zárate.

Medina, J.T. 1887. *Historia del tribunal del Santo Oficio de la Inquisición de Lima, 1569–1820.* 2 vols. Santiago de Chile: Gutenberg

Meléndez, Juan. 1681. *Tesoros verdaderos de las Indias.* Rome: Nicolás Ángel Tinassio

Memorias de los virreyes que han gobernado el Perú durante el tiempo del coloniaje español. 1859. 6 vols. Lima: Librería Central de Felipe Bailly

Mendiburu, Manuel de. 1878–90. *Diccionario histórico-biográfico del Perú.* 8 vols. Lima: Imprenta de J. Francisco Solís

Moreno, Gabriel. 1872. "Elogio del doctor Cosme Bueno." In *Documentos literarios del Perú,* 5–10, ed. Manuel de Odriozola. Lima: Imprenta del Estado

Nolasco Crespo, Pedro. 1791. "Carta escrita a la sociedad por el doctor don Pedro Nolasco Crespo, proponiendo unas nuevas conjeturas sobre el flujo y el reflujo del mar." *Mercurio peruano* 46–47 (12 June): 96–101 and 104–111

Novísima recopilación de las Leyes de España: Dividida en XII libros, en que se reforma la Recopilacion publicada por el Señor Don Felipe II. en el año de 1567, reimpresa últimamente en el de 1804, mandada formar por el Señor Don Carlos IV. 1805. Madrid: n.p.

"Nuevo método para curar la disentería." 1793 *Mercurio peruano* 291 (17 October): 105–7

Numeración generale de todas las personas de ambos sexos, edades y calidades que se ha hecho en la ciudad de Lima. Año de 1700. 1985. Facsimile, ed. Noble David Cook. Lima: COFIDE

Odriozola, Manuel de. 1877. *Documentos literarios del Perú.* Vol. 11. Lima: Imprenta del Estado

Ordenanzas de la sociedad patriótica del monte Pio de los cirujanos del Perú aprobadas por este superior gobierno y real acuerdo de justicia en 12 de marzo de 1800. 1802. Lima: En la Imprenta de la Casa Real de Niños Expósitos

Ordenanças del buen gobierno de la Armada del mar océano de 24 de enero de 1633. 1974 [1678]. Facsimile. Madrid: Instituto histórico de la Marina

Ordenanzas generales de la Armada naval. Part I: Sobre la gobernación militar y marinera de la Armada en general y uso de sus fuerzas en el mar. 1793. Vol. 1. Madrid: En la imprenta de la viuda de don Joachîn de Ibarra.

Origen y descubrimiento de la vaccina. 1802. Trans. Pedro Hernández. Madrid: Benito García.

Ortega y Pimentel, Isidro José. 1764. *Oración comminatoria que, a fin de corregir los excesos de algunos profesores de las artes subalternas a la medicina, dijo el día cuatro de octubre del presente año de 1764, el Doct. D. Isidro Joseph Ortega y Pimentel, catedrático de Método en la Real universidad de San Marcos.* Lima: En la Oficina de la calle de la Encarnación

Ossera y Estella, José Miguel de. 1690. *El físico christiano. PartI: Libro de la entrada a su noble exercicio.* Lima: Luis de Lyra

Pauw, Cornelius de. 1770. *Recherches philosophiques sur les Américains, ou, Mémoires interessants pour servir à l'histoire de l'espèce humaine.* 3 vols. Berlin: n.p.

Petit, Pablo. 1717. *Questiones generales sobre el modo de partear y cuidar a las mujeres que están embarazadas o paridas.* Madrid: Ángel Pascual Rubia

– 1723 *Epístola oficiosa sobre esencia y curación del cáncer, vulgarmente llamado Zaratán.* Lima: Ignacio de Luna

– 1730 *Breve tratado de la enfermedad venerea o mal gálico.* Lima: En la imprenta que está en la Calle Real de Palacio.

Philaletes (pseudonym). 1791. "Carta sobre los maricones." *Mercurio peruano* 94 (27 November): 229–32

– 1793a. "Carta remitida a la sociedad criticando diversos rasgos impresos en el *Mercurio*." *Mercurio peruano* 224–6 (24–28 February and 3 March): 136–55

– 1793b. "Carta escrita a la sociedad en contestación de la disertación apologética impresa en el *Mercurio* núm. 246." *Mercurio peruano* 255–7 (13–20 June): 116–22

Prince, Carlos, ed. 1890. *Lima Antigua: Tipos de antaño*. Lima: Imprenta del Universo

Raynal, Abbé Guillaume-Thomas. 1777. *History of the Settlements and Trade of the Europeans in the East and West Indies*. Vol. 5, trans. by J. Justamond. London: Printed for T. Cadell. [Translation of *Histoire philosophique et politique des deux Indes*. Amsterdam, 1770]

Reclamo al Excmo. Gobierno, del Dr. D. José Indelicato, por denegada justicia: En un decreto del Sr. Jeneral Prefecto de este departamento, fecha 5 del corriente, publicado en el Eco del Norte el 7 del mismo mes, al que siguió el dia despues, en virtud, de una clausula del mismo decreto, una oposicion de la Policia á que el dicho doctor obtuviese el pasaporte que habia pedido para pasar al Ecuador. 1838. Lima: J. Masías

Recopilación de leyes de los Reinos de las Indias. 1681. Vol. 2. Madrid: Julián de Paredes

Recopilación de leyes de los Reinos de las Indias. 1841. 4 Vols. Madrid: Boix, 1841

"Reflexiones históricas y políticas sobre el estado de la población de esta capital, que se acompaña por suplemento." 1791. *Mercurio peruano* 10 (3 February): 90–9

Reflexiones políticas y morales de un descendiente de África a su nación en que manifiesta sus amorosas quejas a los americanos sus hermanos. 1812. Lima: Por Bernardino Ruiz en la Imprenta de los Húerfanos

Refutacion de un informe del doctor don J. Gastañeta, diputado avaluador del gremio de médicos: Al señor jeneral prefecto, dirijido á demonstrar que los profesores de medicina estranjeros deben pagar el maximum de la contribucion sobre este ramo de industria; y que por lo mismo, perteneciendo á esta clase de médicos el doctor don José Indelicato, cualesquiera que sean sus circunstancias particulares, debe ser comprendido entre los que pagan patente de prímera [sic] clase, á pesar de su reclamo; al que, en virtud del dicho informe, se decretó no haber lugar. 1838. Lima: J. Masías

Reglamento Colegio de la Independencia. 1862. In *Colección de leyes, decretos y órdenes publicadas en el Perú desde el año de 1821 hasta 21 de diciembre de 1859.* Vol. 9. Lima: Felipe Bailly

"Resultado del pronóstico y precauciones para el otoño publicados en el *Mercurio peruano* tom. 1, pág. 275." 1791. *Mercurio peruano* 82 (16 October): 121–31

Rivilla Bonet y Pueyo, Joseph [attributed to Pedro Peralta Barnuevo]. 1695. *Desvíos de la naturaleza o tratado del origen de los monstruos.* Lima: En la Imprenta Real

Roque, Abbé de la, ed. 1683. *Journal de médecine ou observations de plus fameux médecins, chirurgiens et anatomistes de l'Europe.* Paris: Chez Fl. Lambert et J. Cusson

Rossi y Rubí, Joseph [under the pseudonym Hesperióphylo]. 1791. "Idea de las congregaciones públicas de los negros bozales." *Mercurio peruano* 48–9 (16–19 June): 112–17 and 120–5

Rowley, William. 1793. *The Rational Practice of Physic.* 4 vols. London: printed for the author; sold by E. Newbery; J. Hand; and to be had at No. 21, Saville-Row

Salinas y Córdova, Buenaventura de. 1957 [1630] *Memorial de las historias del Nuevo Mundo. Pirú.* Lima: Universidad Nacional Mayor de San Marcos

Sigaud de la Fond, Joseph Aignan. 1800 [1781] *Diccionario de las maravillas de la naturaleza: que contiente indagaciones profundas sobre los extravíos de la naturaleza, ecos, evacuaciones, fecundidad, enfermedades, etc.* Madrid: J. Real

Smith, Archibald. 1839. *Peru as It Is: A Residence in Lima, and Other Parts of the Peruvian Republic, comprising an Account of the Social and Physical Features of That Country.* 2 vols. London: Richard Bentley

Sociedad académica de amantes del País. 1793. "Introducción al tomo VII del *Mercurio Peruano.*" *Mercurio peruano* 209–10 (3–6 January): 1–24

Solano, Joaquín. 1818. "Uso del tártaro emético en la epidemia catarral biliosa de Lima." *Gaceta del Gobierno de Lima* 24 (8 April): 184–9

Solórzano Pereyra, Juan de. 1736. *Política Indiana.* 2 vols. Madrid: Por Mateo Sacristán

Stanhope, P. Henry Stanhope. 1830. *Address of Earl Stanhope, President of the Medico-Botanical Society, for the Anniversary Meeting, January 16, 1830.* London: Printed by J. Wilson

Suárez de Ribera, Francisco. 1736. *Manifestación de cien secretos del doctor Juan Curvo Semmedo, experimentados e ilustrados por el doctor Rivera.* Madrid: En la imprenta de Domingo Fernández de Arrojo

Terralla y Landa, Esteban. *See* Ayanque, Simón

Thimeo [pseudonym]. 1791. "Descripción anatómica de un monstruo." *Mercurio peruano* 1 (2 January): 7–8

Unanue, Hipólito [under the pseudonym "Aristio"]. 1791. "Metamorfoses humanas: Noticia de la extraña desfiguración de una niña." *Mercurio peruano* 55 (14 July): 196–8

– [under the pseudonym "Aristio"]. 1792. "Descripción de un ternero bicipite seguida de algunas reflexiones sobre dos monstruos." *Mercurio peruano* 126 (18 March): 183–92

– 1793a. "Decadencia y restauración del Perú." *Mercurio peruano* 218–22 (3–17 February): 82–127

– 1793b. "Indagaciones sobre la disentería y el vicho: Observación primera hecha en el Real anfiteatro anatómico el día 15 del mes presente." *Mercurio peruano* 258 (23 June): 128–31

– 1793c. "Indagaciones sobre la disentería y el vicho: Observación segunda extraída de las que se han hecho en el Real anfiteatro anatómico." *Mercurio peruano* 283 (19 September): 44–5

– 1794. "Discurso que para el establecimiento de unas conferencias clínicas de medicina y cirujía dijo en el Real anfiteatro anatómico el día 18 del presente mes el doctor don Hipólito Unanue." *Mercurio peruano* 371 (24 July): 195–204

– 1806. *Observaciones sobre el clima de Lima y sus influencias en los seres organizados, en especial el hombre.* Lima: En la Imprenta Real de los Huérfanos

– 1808. *Quadro sinoptico de las ciencias, que se ensenaran en el Colegio de Medicina de San Fernando de Lima: que se funda de orden del Excmo. senor virey don Jose Fernando Abascal y Sousa.* Lima: n.p.

Vadillo, Pedro Gago de. 1692 [1632]. *Luz de la verdadera cirujía y discursos de censura de ambas vías y elección de la primera intención curativa y unión de las heridas.* Pamplona: Juan Micol

Valdés, José Manuel. 1791a. "Higiene: Carta dirigida a la sociedad por el despacho del *Mercurio.*" *Mercurio peruano* 45 (5 June): 87–95

– 1791b. "Carta segunda de Erisistrato Svadel relativa a las precauciones que deben observarse en los partos en continuación de las publicadas en el Mercurio número 45." *Mercurio peruano* 102 (25 December): 292–9

– 1792a. "Sobre el veneno animal y sus remedios." *Mercurio peruano* 113–14 (2–5 February): 76–89

– 1792b. "Sobre las utilidades de la anatomía comprobadas con una observación." Mercurio peruano 161 (19 July): 180–9

– 1793. "Disertación médico-quirúrgica en la que se expone metódicamente la curación de la disentería y el uso en ella de las ayudas del aire fijo." *Mercurio peruano* 289–90 (10–13 October): 87–102

– 1807. *Theses medicae quas pro gradu licentiatus obtinendo auspice Deo. Iubente Dilectissimo Carolo IV, favente Excmo. Prorege, et praeside D.D. Hyppolito Unanue.* Lima: Imprenta de los Huérfanos

– 1813. "Oda con motivo de la elección popular del Excmo: Ayuntamiento de esta ciudad, celebrada en el mes de diciembre de 1812, con arreglo a lo prevenido en las constituciones de la monarquía española." *El verdadero peruano* 23 (25 February): 223–8

– 1815a. "Disertación sobre la eficacia del bálsamo de Copayba en las convulsiones de los niños." In *Disertaciones médico-quirúrgicas sobre varios puntos importantes*, 8–42. Madrid: En la imprenta de Sancha

– 1815b. "Disertación sobre una epidemia catarral que se padeció en Lima en el año de 1808." In *Disertaciones médico-quirúrgicas sobre varios puntos importantes*, 43–98. Madrid: En la imprenta de Sancha

– 1815c. "Disertación sobre el cancro uterino que padecen las mujeres en Lima." In *Disertaciones médico-quirúrgicas sobre varios puntos importantes*. 99–152. Madrid: En la imprenta de Sancha

– 1815d. "Reflexiones sobre el mejor método de curar las parótidas y el carbunclo." In *Disertaciones médico-quirúrgicas sobre varios puntos importantes*. 153–79. Madrid: En la imprenta de Sancha

– 1818. "Epidemia: Descripción de la que se padece actualmente en Lima por el D.D. José Manuel Valdés, a petición de dos S.S. respetables." *Gaceta del gobierno de Lima* 18 (10 March): 137–40

– 1822. *La fe de Cristo Triunfante en Lima.* Published under the pseudonym Cristófilo. Lima: Imprenta de J. Masías

– 1825. *Oda: Lima libre y pacífica: Al Excmo. Señor Libertador Simón Bolívar, J.M.V.* Lima: Imprenta del Estado, por J. González

– 1827. *Memoria sobre las enfermedades epidémicas que se padecieron en Lima el año de 1821 estando sitiada por el ejército libertador.* Lima: Imprenta de la Libertad

– 1831. "Testamento de José Manuel Valdés." AGN, Protocolos notariales, José Joaquín Luque [escribano], Protocolo 379 (26 March): 1831856r–866r

– 1833. *Salterio Peruano o paráfrasis de los ciento cincuenta salmos de David, y de algunos cánticos sagrados, en castellano para instrucción y*

piadoso ejercicio de todos los fieles y principalmente de los peruanos.
Lima: Imprenta de J. Masías

– 1835a. *Memoria sobre la disentería, sus causas, prognóstico y curación.*
Lima: Imprenta de la Gaceta

– 1835b. *Al público peruano: El Protomédico general de la República en contestación a la diatriba del D.D. Archibaldo Smith, impresa en los números 38 y 39 del periódico titulado El Regenerador.* Lima: Imprenta de J. Masías

– 1836. *Poesías espirituales, escritas a beneficio y para el uso de las personas sencillas y piadosas.* Lima: Imprenta de J. Masías

– 1838. *Memoria sobre el cólera morbus.* Lima: Imprenta de Eusebio Aranda

– 1840. "Testamento de José Manuel Valdés." AGN, Protocolos notariales, Gerónimo de Villafuerte [escribano], Protocolo 1024 (25 June): 463v–468r

– 1841. "Testamento de José Manuel Valdés." AGN, Protocolos notariales, Gerónimo de Villafuerte [escribano], Protocolo 1024 (30 July): 584v–589v

– 1841. *Dissertatio medica de crisibus et diebus criticis in usum alumnorum collegii medicinae peruanae.* Lima: Imprenta de José Masías

– 1853. "Oda a San Martín." In *Lira patriótica del Perú,* 26–31. Lima: Imprenta de Fernando Velarde

– 1863. [1840]. *Vida admirable del bienaventurado fray Martín de Porres.* Lima: Huerta

– 1871. "Oda a San Martín." In *Parnaso peruano,* ed. José Domingo Cortes, 763–8. Valparaiso: Imprenta Albión de Cox y Taylor

Valdizán, Hermilio. 1927. *La Facultad de Medicina de Lima.* 3 vols. Lima: n.p.

Valle y Caviedes, Juan del. 1984. *Obra completa.* Caracas: Biblioteca Ayacucho

Vargas Machuca, Francisco. 1694. *Oración panegírica al Glorioso Apostol San Bartolomé, Patrón del Hospital Real de pobres negros horros enfermos, viejos e impedidos fundado en esta Nobilísima Ciudad de los Reyes.* Lima: Joseph de Contreras y Alvadado

Velasco, Diego de, and Francisco Villaverde. 1763. *Curso teórico práctico de cirujía en que se continenen los más célebres descubrimientos modernos.* Madrid: Joachim Ibarra

Voltaire [François-Marie Arouet]. 1829 [1764]. *Dictionnaire Philosophique.*
Vol. 6. Paris: Chez Lequien Fils
Von Tschudi, J.J. 1854. *Travels in Peru, on the Coast, in the Sierra, across
the Cordilleras, and the Andes, into the Primeval Forests.* New York:
A.S. Barnes and Co.
Winslow, Jacques-Benigne. 1732. *Exposition anatomique de la structure
du corps humain.* Paris: Guillaume Desprez et Jean Desessartz

MODERN SOURCES

Acree, William G., Jr., and Alex Borucki. 2010. *Jacinto Ventura de Molina:
Los caminos de la escritura negra en el Río de la Plata.* Foreword by
George R. Andrews. Madrid: Iberoamericana
Aguirre, Carlos. 1993. *Agentes de su propia libertad: Los esclavos de
Lima y la desintegración de la esclavitud: 1821–1854.* Lima: Pontificia
Universidad Católica del Perú, Fondo Editorial
Andrews, George R. 2004. *Afro-Latin America, 1800–2000.* Oxford:
Oxford University Press
– 2010. *Blackness in the White Nation: A History of Afro-Uruguay.*
Chapel Hill: University of North Carolina Press
Anna, Timothy E. 1975. "The Peruvian Declaration of Independence:
Freedom by Coercion." *Journal of Latin American Studies* 7, no. 2:
221–48
– 1979. *The Fall of the Royal Government in Peru.* Lincoln: University of
Nebraska Press
Aragón Espeso, M. 2009. "Los sanitarios de la armada en el siglo XVIII."
Sanidad militar: Revista de sanidad de las Fuerzas armadas de España
65, no. 2: 117–31
Atug F., F. Akay, U. Aflay, H. Sahin, and A. Yalinkaya. 2005. "Delivery of
Dead Fetus from inside Urinary Bladder with Uterine Perforation: Case
Report and Review of Literature." *Urology* 65, no. 4: 797e11–797e12
Bancroft-Livingston, George. 1956. "Louise de la Vallière and the Birth of
the Man-Midwife." *BJOG: An International Journal of Obstetrics and
Gynaecology* 63, no. 2: 261–7
Barbagelata, José. 1945. "Apuntes históricos sobre el desarrollo urbano de
Lima." *Evolución urbana de Lima*, eds. Juan Bromley and José Barbage-
lata. Lima: Lumen

Barrera-Osorio, Antonio. 2006. *Experiencing Nature: The Spanish American Empire and the Early Scientific Revolution.* Austin: Texas University Press

Barvosa, Edwina. 2008. *Wealth of Selves: Multiple Identities, Mestiza Consciousness, and the Subject of Politics.* College Station: Texas A & M University Press

Behrend-Martinez, Edward. 2005. "Manhood and the Neutered Body in Early Modern Spain." *Journal of Social History* 38, no. 4: 1073–93

Belaunde, Víctor Andrés. 1987. "El debate constitucional. In Obras completas, vol. 4. Lima: Comisión nacional del centenario de Víctor Andrés Belaunde

Bernard, Carmen. 2003. "Entre pueblo y plebe: Patriotas, pardos, africanos en Argentina (1790–1852)." In *Blacks, Coloureds, and National Identity in Nineteenth-Century Latin America,* ed. Nancy P. Naro, 60–80. London: Institute of Latin American Studies

Bifano, Claudio, and Guillermo Whittembury. 2007. "The First Publication of the New Chemistry in America in *Mercurio peruano* (1792) by Joseph Coquette." *Interciencia* 32, no. 4: 281–8

Blanchard, Peter. 1992. *Slavery and Abolition in Early Republican Peru.* Wilmington, DE: SR Books

– 2008. *Under the Flags of Freedom: Slave Soldiers and the Wars of Independence in Spanish South America.* Pittsburgh: University of Pittsburgh Press

Bowser, Frederick P. 1974. *The African Slave in Colonial Peru, 1524–1650.* Standford: Stanford University Press

Bronner, Fred. 1956. "José de la Riva-Agüero (1885–1944), Peruvian Historian." *Hispanic American Historical Review* 36, no. 4: 490–502

Burke, Michael E. 1977. *The Royal College of San Carlos: Surgery and Spanish Medical Reform in the Late Eighteenth Century.* Durham: Duke University Press

Burshatin, Israel. 1998. "Interrogating Hermaphroditism in Sixteenth-Century Spain." In *Hispanisms and Homosexualities,* ed. Robert McKee Irwin and Silvia Mollow, 3–18. Durham: Duke University Press

Bustios Romaní, Carlos. 2004. *400 años de la salud pública en el Perú (1533–1933).* Lima: Fondo Editorial de la UNMSM-CONCYTEC

Busto Duthurburu, José Antonio del. 2006. *San Martín de Porras.* Lima: Pontificia Universidad Católica del Perú

Cahill, David. 1995. "Financing Health Care in the Viceroyalty of Peru: The Hospitals of Lima in the Late Colonial Period." *The Americas* 52, no. 2: 123–54

Campos Díez, María Soledad. 1996. "El Protomedicato en la administración central de la Monarquía hispánica." *Dynamis: Acta hispanica ad medicinae scientiarumque historiam illustrandam* 16: 43–58

Cañizares-Esguerra, Jorge. 2006. *Nature, Empire, and Nation: Explorations of the History of Science in the Iberian World.* Standford: Standford University Press

Cañizares-Esguerra, Jorge, and Marcos Cueto. 2002. "Latin American Science: The Long View." *NACLA Report on the Americas* 35, no. 5: 18–22

Carrera, Magali. 2003. *Imagining Identity in New Spain: Race, Lineage and the Colonial Body in Portraiture and Casta Paintings.* Austin: University of Texas Press

Castleman, Bruce. 2001. "Social Climbers in a Colonial Mexican City: Individual Mobility within the Sistema de Castas in Orizaba, 1777–1791." *Colonial Latin American Review* 10, no. 2: 229–49

Clement, Jean-Pierre. 1979. "Índices del *Mercurio peruano*." *Fénix: Revista de la Biblioteca nacional del Perú* 26–7:5–234

– *El Mercurio peruano 1790–1795.* 1997. Vol. 1. Frankfurt: Vervuert-Iberoamericana

Cornejo, Andrés Herrera. 2006. *El genio de "El murciélago": Manuel Atanasio Fuentes y sus grabados costumbristas de Lima de 1850.* Lima: Instituto Eugenio Courret

Cruz-Coke Madrid, Ricardo. 1995. *Historia de la medicina chilena.* Santiago de Chile: Editorial Andrés Bello

Cunningham, Andrew. 1989. "Thomas Sydenham: Epidemics, Experiment, and the 'Good Old Cause.'" *The Medical Revolution of the Seventeenth Century.* Eds. Roger French and Andrew Wear. Cambridge: Cambridge University Press

Cussen, Celia L. 2005. "The Search for Idols and Saints in Colonial Peru: Linking Extirpation and Beatification." *Hispanic American Historical Review* 85, no. 3: 417–48

Dager Alva, Joseph. 2001. "Hipólito Unanue en el *Mercurio peruano*." *Revista de historia de América* 128: 97–121

Deans-Smith, Susan. 2005. "Creating the Colonial Subject: Casta Paintings, Collectors, and Critics in Eighteenth-Century Mexico and Spain." *Colonial Latin American Review* 14, no. 2: 169–204

Dejo Bustios, Hugo A. 2008. *Apuntes de salud y medicina del Perú antiguo*. Lima: Nóstica editorial.

Delgado Matallana, Gustavo, and Miguel Rabí Chara. 2006. *Evolución histórica de la facultad de medicina de San Fernando*. Lima: UNMSM

Delgar, Martín.1980 [1800]. *Libro de medicina y cirugía para el uso de los pobres con su recetario al final*. Lima: UNMSM, Seminario de Historia Rural Andina

De Vos, Paula S. 2006. "Research, Development, and Empire: State Support of Science in the Later Spanish Empire." *Colonial Latin American Review* 15, no. 1: 55–79

Few, Martha. 2007. "That Monster of Nature": Gender, Sexuality, and the Medicalization of a 'Hermaphrodite' in Late Colonial Guatemala." *Ethnohistory: The Bulletin of the Ohio Valley Historic Indian Conference* 54, no. 1: 159–76

Fields, Sherry. 2008. *Pestilence and Headcolds: Encountering Illness in Colonial Mexico*. New York: Columbia University Press

Fisher, Andrew B., and Matthew D. O'Hara. 2009. *Imperial Subjects: Race and Identity in Colonial Latin America*. Durham: Duke University Press

Flores Galindo, Alberto. 1991. *La ciudad sumergida: Aristocracia y plebe en Lima, 1760–1830*. Lima: Editorial Horizonte

Gamio Palacios, Fernando. 2005. *La municipalidad de Lima y la emancipación (1821)*. Lima: Municipalidad de Lima

García Cáceres, Uriel. 1999. *Juan del Valle y Caviedes, cronista de la medicina: historia de la medicina en el Perú en la segunda mitad del siglo XVII*. Lima: Banco Central de Reserva del Perú.

– 2002. "El cólera en la Historia de la medicina social peruana: Comentarios sobre un decreto precursor." *Revista peruana de medicina experimental y salud pública* 19, no. 2: 97–101

Gargurevich, Juan. 1999. "Manuel Atanasio Fuentes: Un limeño del siglo XIX." *Letras* 97–8: 61–80

Garofalo, Leo J. 2006. "Conjuring with Coca and the Inca: The Andeanization of Lima's Afro-Peruvian Ritual Specialists, 1580–1690." *The Americas* 63, no. 1: 53–80

Gerbi, Antonello. 2010. *The Dispute of the New World: The History of a Polemic, 1750–1900*. Translated by Jeremy Moyle. Pittsburgh: University of Pittsburgh Press

Gittinger, Georgianna Simmons. 1945. "Miguel Tafur – Protomédico." *Bulletin of the History of Medicine* 17: 315–19

Glick, Thomas. 1991. "Science and Independence in Latin America (with Special Reference to New Granada)." *The Hispanic American Historical Review* 71, no. 2: 307–34

Goicoetxea Marcaida, Ángel. 1989. "Juan José Tafalla y Nabasques, botánico olvidado de la Ilustración." *Príncipe de Viana* (Pamplona) 50, no. 188: 641–7

Gómez Ocaña, J. 1912. "El doctor Bartolomé Hidalgo de Agüero, renombrado el Pareo español: Breve noticias de su vida y obras." *Bulletin Hispanique* 14: 96–100

González, Ondina E. 2007. "Introduction: Children of the Empire." In *Raising an Empire: Children in Early Modern Iberia and Colonial Latin America*, ed. Ondina E. Gonzálex and Bianca Premo. Albuquerque: University of New Mexico Press

Goodwin, Stefan. 2009. *Africa in Europe: Interdependencies, Relocations, and Globalization*. Vol. 2. Lanham: Lexington Books

Gorbach, Frida. 2000. "Mujeres, monstruos e impresiones en la medicina mexicana del siglo XIX." *Relaciones* (Revista del Colegio de Michoacán) 21, no. 81: 41–55

Griffiths, Nicolas. 1999. "Andean Curanderos and Their Repressors: The Persecution of Native Healing in Late Seventeenth- and Early Eighteenth-Century Peru." In *Spiritual Encounters: Interactions between Christianity and Native Religions in Colonial America*, eds. Nicholas Griffiths and Fernando Cervantes, 185–97. Lincoln: University of Nebraska Press

Hamnet, Brian R. 2000. "La política contrarrevolucionaria del Virrey Abascal: Perú, 1806–1816." *Serie historia* 18 [documento de trabajo 112]. Lima: Instituto de Estudios peruanos

Hanafi, Zakiya. 2000. *The Monster in the Machine: Magic, Medicine, and the Marvelous in the Time of the Scientific Revolution*. Durham, NC: Duke University Press

Herrera Cornejo, H. Andrés. 2006. *El genio de "El Murciélago": Manuel Atanasio Fuentes y sus grabados costumbristas de Lima de 1850*. Lima: Instituto Fotográfico Eugenio Courret

Herrera, Fortunato. 1937. "Juan Tafalla, ilustre botanico espanol: Primer catedratico de fitografia de la Universidad de San Marcos." *Revista de ciencias* (Lima) 39: 47–60

Hibbard, Bryan M. 2000. *The Obstetrician's Armamentarium: Historical Obstetric Instruments and Their Inventors*. San Anselmo, CA: Norman Publishers

Higgins, James. 2005. *Lima: A Cultural History*. Oxford: Oxford University Press

Hinton, Robert. 2004. "Bahia and the Academic Tourist." In *Monuments of the Black Atlantic: Slavery and Memory*, eds. Joanne M. Braxton and María Diedrich, 9–18. Münster: LIT Verlag

Horswell, Michael J. 2005. *Decolonizing the Sodomite: Queer Tropes of Sexuality in Colonial Andean Culture*. Austin: University of Texas Press

Hünefeldt, Christine. 1994. *Paying the Price of Freedom: Family and Labor among Lima's Slaves, 1800–1854*. Berkeley: University of California Press.

Iwasaki Cauti, Fernando. 1994. "Fray Martín de Porras: Santo, ensalmador y sacamuelas." *Colonial Latin American Review* 3, nos. 1–2: 159–84

Jackson, Richard L. 1997. *Black Writers and the Hispanic Canon*. New York: Twayne Publishers

Jiménez Borja, José. 1962. *Don José de la Riva-Agüero y Osma: Notas sobre su vida, obra y estilo*. Lima, Perú: PUCP

Jouve Martín, José Ramón. 2004. "En olor de santidad: Cultos locales y política de canonizaciones en el Virreinato del Perú". *Colonial Latin American Review* 13, no. 2: 181–98

– 2005. *Esclavos de la ciudad letrada: Esclavitud, escritura y colonialismo en Lima, 1650–1700*. Lima: Instituto de Estudios peruanos

– 2007. "Public Ceremonies and Mulatto Identity in Viceregal Lima: A Colonial Reenactment of the Fall of Troy (1631)." *Colonial Latin American Review* 16, no. 2: 179–201

– 2009. "Death, Gender, and Writing: Testaments of Women of African Origin in Seventeenth-Century Lima (1651–1666)." In *Afro-Latino Voices: Narratives from the Early Modern Ibero-Atlantic World, 1550–1808*, ed. Kathryn McKnight and Leo Garofalo, 105–25. Indianapolis: Hackett

Katzew, Ilona. 1996. *New World Orders: Casta Painting and Colonial Latin America*. New York: Americas Society Art Gallery

– 2004. *Casta Painting: Images of Race in Eighteenth-Century Mexico*. New Haven: Yale University Press

King, James F. 1951. "The Case of José Ponciano de Ayarza: A Document on *Gracias al Sacar*." *Hispanic American Historical Review* 31, no. 4: 640–57

– 1953a. "The Colored Castes and American Representation in the Cortes of Cadiz." *Hispanic American Historical Review* 33, no. 1: 33–64.

– 1953b. "A Royalist View of the Colored Castes in the Venezuelan Wars of Independence." *Hispanic American Historical Review* 33, no. 4: 526–37

Knight, Frnaklin. 2003. "Blacks and the Forging of National Identity in the Caribbean, 1840–1900." In *Coloureds and National Identity in Nineteenth-Century Latin America*, ed. Nancy P. Naro, 81–94. London: Institute of Latin American Studies

Laguerre, Michel. 1988. *Afro-Caribbean Folk Medicine*. Massachusetts: Bergin & Garvey

Langer, Erick D. 2009. *Expecting Pears from an Elm Tree: Franciscan Missions on the Chiriguano Frontier in the Heart of South America, 1830–1949*. Durham: Duke University Press

Lanning, John Tate. 1940. *Academic Culture in the Spanish Colonies*. Oxford: Oxford University Press

– 1969. "The Illicit Practice of Medicine in the Spanish Empire in America." In *Homenaje a Don José María de la Peña Camara*, 143–79. Madrid: Ediciones José Porrua Turanzas

– 1985. *The Royal Protomedicato: The Regulation of the Medical Professions in the Spanish Empire*, ed. John Jay TePaske. Durham: Duke University Press

Lastres, Juan B. 1943. *Vida y obra del Dr. Miguel Tafur*. Lima: Imprenta americana

– 1951a. *La medicina en el virreinato*. Book 2 of *Historia de la medicina peruana*. In *Historia de la universidad*, vol. 5, ed. Luis Antonio Eguiguren. Lima: Santa María

– 1951b. *La medicina en la república*. Book 3 of *Historia de la medicina peruana*. In *Historia de la universidad*, vol. 5, ed. Luis Antonio Eguiguren. Lima: Santa María

– 1955. "El doctor José Manuel Dávalos (1758–1821)." *Documenta: Revista de la sociedad peruana de historia* 3, no. 1: 155–82

Lewis, Laura A. 2003. *Hall of Mirrors: Power, Witchcraft, and Caste in Colonial Mexico*. Durham: Duke University Press

Lindeboom, Gerrit Arie. 1970. "Boerhaave's Impact on Medicine." In *Boerhaave and His Time*, ed. Gerrit Arie Lindeboom, 31–9. Leiden: Brill

Lockhart, James. 1994. *Spanish Peru, 1532–1560: A Social History*. 2nd edition. Madison: University of Wisconsin Press

López Martínez, Héctor. 1993. *El protomédico limeño José Manuel Valdés*. Lima: Dirección de intereses marítimos, Fondo de Publicaciones

Lossio, Jorge. 2006. "British Medicine in the Peruvian Andes: The Travels of Archibald Smith, M.D. (1820–1870)." *História, Ciências, Saúde – Manguinhos* 13, no. 4: 833–50

Luis, William. 1990. *Literary Bondage: Slavery in Cuban Narrative.* Austin: University of Texas Press

Luis, William. 2007. *Autobiografía del esclavo poeta y otros escritos.* Madrid: Iberoamericana

McEvoy Carreras, Carmen. 2002. "Seríamos excelentes vasallos, y nunca ciudadanos: Prensa republicana y cambio social en Lima (1791–1822)." In *Sobre el Perú: Homenaje a José A. de la Puente Candamo,* vol. 2, 825–62. Lima: PUCP

McKinley, Michelle A. 2010. "Such Unsightly Unions Could Never Result in Holy Matrimony": Mixed-Status Marriages in Seventeenth-Century Colonial Lima." *Yale Journal of Law and the Humanities* 22, no. 2: 217–55

– 2012. "Till Death Do Us Part: Testamentary Manumision in Seventeenth-Century Lima, Peru." *Slavery and Abolition* 33, no. 3: 381–401

McPheeters, D.W. 1955. "The Distinguished Peruvian Scholar Cosme Bueno 1711–1798." *Hispanic American Historical Review* 35, no. 4: 484–91

Mark, Catherine. 2009. "The World's First Immunization Campaign: The Spanish Smallpox Vaccine Expedition, 1803–1813." *Bulletin of the History of Medicine* 83, no. 1: 63–94

Martínez Riaza, Ascensión. 1982. "Los orígenes del periodismo doctrinario en Perú: El caso conflictivo de 'El Peruano.'" *Quinto centenario* 3: 109–34

Meléndez, Mariselle. 2006. "Patria, Criollos, and Blacks: Imagining the Nation in the Mercurio peruano, 1791–1795." *Colonial Latin American Review* 15, no. 2: 207–27

– 2011. *Deviant and Useful Citizens: The Cultural Production of the Female Body in Eighteenth-Century Peru.* Nashville: Vanderbilt University Press

Menéndez Pelayo, Marcelino. 1948. *Historia de la poesía hispanoamericana.* Edición nacional de las obras completas de Menéndez Pelayo. Vol. 28. Madrid: Consejo Superior de Investigaciones Científicas

Morán Ramos, Luis Daniel. 2008. *Reformistas, fidelistas y contrarrevolucionarios: Prensa, poder y discurso político en Lima durante las Cortes de Cádiz (1810–1814).* Tesis de Licenciatura. Universidad Nacional Mayor de San Marcos. Lima

– 2010. "De la reforma a la contrarrevolución: Prensa y discurso político
en la coyuntura de las cortes de Cádiz en el Perú." *Temas americanistas*
24: 107–30

Mott, Luiz. 2005. "Filhos de Abraão e de Sodoma: Cristãos-novos homos-
sexuais nos tempos da Inquisição." In *Ensaios sobre a intolerância: Inquisição, marranismo e anti-semitismo*, 2nd edition, ed. Lina Gorenstein
and Maria Luiza Tucci Carneiro, 25–66. Sao Paulo: Associaçao Editorial
Humanitas

Naro, Nancy Priscilla. 2003. *Blacks, Coloureds, and National Identity in
Nineteenth-Century Latin America*. London: Institute of Latin American
Studies

Newson, Linda A. 2006. "Medical Practice in Early Colonial Spanish
America: A Prospectus." *Bulletin of Latin American Research* 25, no. 3:
367–91

Nemesio Vargas, M. 1910. *Historia del Perú Independiente*. Vol. 4. Lima:
Imprenta del Lucero

Núñez Hague, Estuardo. 1998. *Manuel Atanasio Fuentes, Marco A. de la
Fuente, Aureliano Villarán: Tradiciones Desconocidas*. Lima: Instituto
latinoamericano de cultura y desarrollo

Nwankwo, Ifeoma Kiddoe. 2005. *Black Cosmopolitanism: Racial Consciousness and Transnational Identity in the Nineteenth-Century Americas*. Philadelphia: University of Pennsylvania Press

O'Phelan Godoy, Scarlett. 2002. "Ciudadanía y etnicidad en las Cortes de
Cádiz." *Elecciones* 1: 165–85

Orrego Penagos, Juan Luis. 2009. "La contrarrevolución del virrey Abascal: Lima, 1806–1816." *Procesos: Revista ecuatoriana de Historia* 29,
no. 1: 93–112

O'Toole, Rachel S. 2012. *Bound Lives: Africans, Indians, and the Making
of Race in Colonial Peru*. Pittsburgh: University of Pittsburgh Press

Pamo Reyna, Oscar. 2000. "Publicaciones periódicas peruanas." In
Historia de la medicina peruana en el siglo XX, vol. 2, ed. Oswaldo
Salaverry García, comp. Gustavo Delgado Matallana, 1369–78. Lima:
Universidad Mayor de San Marcos

– 2009. "Los médicos próceres de la independencia del Perú." *Acta
médica peruana* 26, no. 1: 58–66

Paniagua Corazao. 2003. *Los orígenes del gobierno representativo en
Perú: Las elecciones (1809–1826)*. Lima. Pontificia Universidad Católica
del Perú

Park, Katharine, and Lorraine J. Daston. 1981. "Unnatural Conceptions: The Study of Monsters in Sixteenth- and Seventeenth-Century France and England." *Past and Present* 92, no. 1: 20–54

Paz-Soldán, Carlos Enrique. 1942. *José Manuel Valdés, 1767–1843*. Lima: Imp. "Lux"

Peralta Ruiz, Víctor. 2008. "El impacto de las Cortes de Cádiz en el Perú: Un balance historiográfico." *Revista de Indias* 68, no. 242: 67–96

– 2011. "La pluma contra las Cortes y el Trono. La prensa y el desmontaje del liberalismo hispánico en el Perú, 1821–1824." *Revista de Indias* 71, no. 253: 729–58

Pérez Cantó, Pilar. 1982. "La población de Lima en el siglo XVIII." *Boletín americanista* 32: 383–407

Poska, Allyson. 2010. "Babies on Board: Women, Children, and Imperial Policy in the Spanish Empire." *Gender and History* 22, no. 2: 269–83

Premo, Bianca. 2005a. " 'Misunderstood Love': Children and Wet Nurses, Creoles, and Kings in Lima's Enlightenment." *Colonial Latin American Review* 14, no. 2: 231–61

– 2005b. *Children of the Father King: Youth, Authority, and Legal Minority in Colonial Lima*. Chapel Hill: University of North Carolina Press

Price, Robin. 1979. "Spanish Medicine in the Golden Age." *Journal of the Royal Society of Medicine* 72: 864–74

Proceso de beatificación de fray Martín de Porres. 1960. Palencia: Secretariado Martín de Porres

Rabí Chara, Miguel. 2001. *El hospital de San Bartolomé de Lima (1646–2000): La protección y asistencia de la gente de color*. Lima: GRAHUER, 2001

– 2006a. "La formación de médicos y cirujanos durante los siglos XVI a XIX: Las escuelas prácticas de medicina y cirugía en el Perú." *Anales de la Facultad de Medicina* 67, no. 2: 173–83

– 2006b. *La vida y la obra singular de un cirujano criollo. Primer defensor de su gremio en el Perú: José Pastor de Larrinaga (1758–ca.1821)*. Lima: Hospital nacional docente madre niño "San Bartolomé"

Ramsey, Matthew. 1992. "The Popularization of Medicine in France, 1650–1900." In *The Popularization of Medicine, 1650–1850*, ed. Roy Porter, 97–133. London: Routledge

– 1994. "Academic Medicine and Medical Industrialism: The Regulation of Secret Remedies in Nineteenth-Century France." In *French Medical*

Culture in the Nineteenth Century, ed. Ann LaBerge and Mordechai Feingold, 25–32. Amsterdam: Rodopi B.V.

"Reseña histórica de la Provincia de San Juan Bautista del Perú." 2012. Frailes dominicos en el Perú. (accessed 2 April 2012). http://peru.op.org/historia-de-la-provincia.html

Restall, Matthew. 2000. "Black Conquistadors: Armed Africans in Early Spanish America." *The Americas* 57, no. 2: 171–205

"Review IX: History of Medicine in Spain". 1861. *British and Foreign Medico-Chirurgical Review* 27 (April): 198–219

Riera Palmero, Juan Bautista. 2000. *Protomedicato, humanismo y medicina en Castilla*. Valladolid: Universidad de Valladolid

Rodríguez Merino, José María. 1990. "Biomecanicismo, bioclima y biopoítica en la medicina ilustrada peruana." LLULL 13: 517–37

Rodríguez-Sala, María Luisa. 2011. "Cruzar el Atlantico al servicio de la enfermedad: Los cirujanos en las 'Flotas de los galeones' o de 'Tierra Firme,' Siglo XVII" (accessed 6 February 2011). http://www.iis.unam.mx/biblioteca/pdf/rodri_sala03.pdf

Romero, Fernando. 1942. "José Manuel Valdés, Great Peruvian Mulatto." *Phylon* 3.3: 296–319.

Rousseau, George Sebastian, and David Boyd Haycock. 2003. "Coleridge's Choleras: Cholera Morbus, Asiatic Cholera, and Dysentery in Early Nineteenth-Century England." *Bulletin of the History of Medicine* 77, no. 2: 298–331

Rutter-Jenson, Chole. 2007. "La transformación transatlantica de la monja alferez." *Revista de estudios sociales* 28: 86–95

Silverblatt, Irene. 2004. *Modern Inquisitions: Peru and the Colonial Origins of the Civilized World*. Durham: Duke University Press

Simmons, John Galbraith. 2002. *Doctors and Discoveries: Lives That Created Today's Medicine*. Boston: Houghton Mifflin

Sobrevilla Perea, Natalia. 2009. "Batallas por la legitimidad: Constitucionalismo y conflicto político en el Perú del siglo XIX (1812–1860)." *Revista de Indias* 69, no. 246: 101–28

Soulodre-LaFrance, Renée. 2010. "What Is in a body? Hermaphrodites and Late Colonial Order in Nueva Granada." *La habana elegante* 48 (accessed 7 March 2011). http://www.habanaelegante.com/index.html

Sweet, James H. 2011. *Domingos Alvares, African Healing, and the Intellectual History of the Atlantic World*. Chapel Hill: University of North Carolina Press

Thomson, Sinclair. 2011. "Was There Race in Colonial Latin America? Identifying Selves and Others in the Insurgent Andes." In *Histories of Race and Racism: The Andes and Mesoamerica from Colonial Times to the Present*, ed. Laura Gotkowitz, 72–93. Durham: Duke University Press

Twinam, Ann. 2009. "Purchasing Whiteness: Conversations on the Essence of Pardo-ness and Mulatto-ness at the End of Empire." In *Imperial Subjects: Race and Identity in Colonial Latin America*, ed. Andrew B. Fisher and Matthew D. O'Hara, 141–66. Durham, NC: Duke University Press

Valdizán, Hermilio. 1927–29. *La Facultad de Medicina de Lima*. 3 vols. Lima: n.p.

Van Deusen, Nancy E. 1999. "The 'Alienated' Body: Slaves and Castas in the Hospital de San Bartolomé in Lima, 1680 to 1700." *The Americas* 56, no. 1: 1–30

– 2004. *The Souls of Purgatory: The Spiritual Diary of a Seventeenth-Century Afro-Peruvian Mystic, Ursula de Jesus*. Albuquerque: University of New Mexico Press

Vargas Ugarte, Rubén. 1943. "La biblioteca medica de D. Jose Manuel Davalos." *Cuadernos del Instituto de investigaciones historicas de la Universidad Catolica* 5: 325–42

Vidal Ortega, Antonino. 2002. *Cartagena de Indias y la región histórica del Caribe, 1580–1640*. Sevilla: CSIC, Escuela de Estudios Hispano-Americanos.

Villegas Páucar, Samuel A. 2012. "La participación de Dionisio Inca Yupanqui en las Cortes de Cádiz, 1810–1814." *Actas del II Congreso Internacional hacia el Bicentenario: 200 años de vida republicana. Balance y perspectivas*. Lima: Universidad Mayor de San Marcos. http://vrinvestigacion.unmsm.edu.pe/eventosVRI/taller/2010/Bicentenario/Ponencias_II_Congreso_Bicentenario/SamuelVillegas_Artic_Dionisio_Inca_Yupanqui.pdf

Voeks, Robert. 1993. "African Medicine and Magic in the Americas." *Geographical Review* 83, no. 1: 66–78

Vollendorf, Lisa. 2005. *The Lives of Women: A New History of Inquisitional Spain*. Nashville: Vanderbilt University Press

Wade, Peter. 1997. *Race and Ethnicity in Latin America*. Chicago: Pluto Press

Walker, Charles F. 2008. *Shaky Colonialism: The 1746 Earthquake-*

Tsunami in Lima, Peru, and Its Long Aftermath. Durham: Duke University Press

Warren, Adam. 2004. "Piety and Danger: Popular Ritual, Epidemics, and Medical Reforms Lima, 1750–1860." PH.D. dissertation. University of California, San Diego

– 2009. "An Operation for Evangelization: Friar Francisco González Laguna, the Cesarean Section, and Fetal Baptism in Late Colonial Peru." *Bulletin of the History of Medicine* 83, no. 4: 647–75

– 2010. *Medicine and Politics in Colonial Peru: Population Growth and the Bourbon Reforms*. Pittsburgh: Pittsburgh University Press

Weaver, Karol K. 2006. *Medical Revolutionaries: The Enslaved Healers of Eighteenth-Century Saint Domingue*. Urbana and Chicago: University of Illinois Press

Woodham, John E. 1964. "Hipolito Unanue and the Enlightenment in Peru." PH.D. dissertation. Duke University, Durham.

– 1970. "The Influence of Hipólito Unanue on Peruvian Medical Science, 1789–1820: A Reappraisal." *Hispanic American Historical Review* 50, no. 4: 693–714

~

Index